# More Than Dispensing,

## a handbook on providing pharmaceutical service to long-term care facilities

Principal author and project director:
Cyrelle K. Gerson, M.S.

Contributing authors:
K. Scott Carruthers, Pharm.D.
Jean Paul Gagnon, Ph.D.
Richard P. Penna, Pharm.D.
Bruce R. Siecker, Ph.D.

Published by the American Pharmaceutical Association
—the national professional society of pharmacists

In addition to "More Than Dispensing," the APhA Academy of Pharmacy Practice Section on Long-Term Care has available a number of other LTC-related publications and services. For more information on these activities, contact:

Cyrelle K. Gerson
Professional Affairs Division
American Pharmaceutical Association
2215 Constitution Ave., N.W.
Washington, DC 20037
(202) 628-4410

**More Than Dispensing**—a handbook on providing pharmaceutical service to long-term care facilities was developed and prepared by Cyrelle K. Gerson, K. Scott Carruthers, Jean Paul Gagnon, Richard P. Penna, and Bruce R. Siecker, with assistance from the APhA Academy of Pharmacy Practice Section on Long-Term Care.

Published by the American Pharmaceutical Association—the national professional society of pharmacists

Cyrelle K. Gerson, Project Director
Nicolette Triantafellu, Editorial Assistant
© 1980, American Pharmaceutical Association, all rights reserved.
Library of Congress Number 80-65958
ISBN 0-917330-31-5

# CONTENTS

# Preface

When launching into a new venture, like taking a trip to an unfamiliar place, or looking for a new route to an old, familiar spot, you need a road map to show you the way. The contents of this book are arranged as a "map" of the thoughts and questions which you may ponder when initiating or reviewing pharmaceutical service for a long-term care facility. These thoughts and questions are arranged stepwise to help you map your course to providing service.

No book can dictate *how* you should provide service. Each situation is unique. You must determine the characteristics of your situation and the best solution to your problems. In this book, we have attempted to help you pose the questions you need to ask and point you in the right direction. We will analyze the steps in providing service. The advantage of such an analysis is that it is not limited to one situation. It can help you evaluate service whether you are an "old pro" or a newcomer. It will help you to ask all the questions you need to ask and in the right order.

The statements and questions in each chapter represent areas that you may have considered in establishing and providing service. The subheadings indicate the section to which you should refer for more information on each area and guidance in answering these questions. You may wish to read this book from beginning to end, but you more likely will refer to the sections which can help you to solve your unique problems.

A book of this type requires the cooperative effort and assistance of many people. An advisory panel reviewed the book from beginning to end. The advisory panel members were K. Scott Carruthers, Alan Cheung, Paul F. Davis, Monroe D. Lipman, Jeffrey Stauffer, and Susan Torrico.

Samuel H. Kalman, APhA director of education, and Richard P. Penna, APhA director of professional affairs, helped to develop the initial concept and outline for the book. Dr. Penna also reviewed every step of preparation of the draft.

Several pharmacists provided consultation on specific forms or sections of the book. They were Frank Albright, Kathleen Fon, Leonard Grossman, Joel Kahn, Robert Leventhal, John Ricci, and Suzanne Vlach. Selected portions of the book were reviewed by Carl Roberts, APhA associate general counsel.

The section on policy and procedure manuals was adapted from workshop materials prepared by Sara J. White.

In addition to those already mentioned, the final draft of the book was reviewed by James W. Cooper, Samuel W. Kidder, and Robert L. Snively.

Also included are the ideas and suggestions of many pharmacists concerned with long-term care, particularly members of the APhA Academy of Pharmacy Practice Section on Long Term Care. They reflect practice innovations that have occurred in diverse geographic locations.

The experience in long-term care of those who have contributed in some way to this project adds up to several hundred years. I am grateful to all of them for sharing this wealth of experience so that others can benefit from it.

March 1980
American Pharmaceutical Association
Washington, D.C.

Cyrelle K. Gerson
Director of Special Projects
Professional Affairs Division

# Introduction

What is the purpose of this book?

Pharmacists who serve long-term care facilities should know in detail what services to offer, how, and why. They need this information in a way that can be readily applied to practice.

The results of a 1969 survey[1] of long-term care pharmacists concluded:

*A very critical problem has been that the pharmacist did not know the needs and internal procedures of the nursing home. When confronted with the offer of being a pharmaceutical consultant, many were at a loss as to what was expected of them.*

Pharmacists' knowledge about pharmaceutical service to long-term care facilities has changed substantially since 1969; however, it is still true that pharmacists need to know what a long-term care facility is, how it fits into the total health care spectrum, and what its characteristics and problems are, in order to provide a useful service. Pharmacists should also be aware of how pharmaceutical service fits into that set of services that comprise long-term care.

## BACKGROUND INFORMATION (Chapters 1-4)

Chapter 1 describes what long-term care is, how it fits into the health care spectrum, and service delivery issues associated with long-term care. Chapters 2, 3, and 4 detail pharmaceutical services and how they are provided and are organized similarly.

Chapter 2 offers an overview of the basic responsibilities of pharmaceutical service; Chapter 3 discusses dispensing services; and Chapter 4 covers nondispensing services. The pertinent activities are categorized according to a scheme developed in Chapter 2. The discussions in Chapters 3 and 4 also follow this scheme. The discussion of each category is introduced with a highlighted list of pharmacist's responsibilities, followed by general or specific procedures for carrying out those responsibilities.

Items for the lists of responsibilities were adapted from the American Pharmaceutical Association-American Association of Colleges of Pharmacy Standards of Practice for the Profession of Pharmacy with appropriate additions from the federal long-term care regulations for Medicare and Medicaid, standards of the Joint Commission on the Accreditation of Hospitals, and other applicable long-term care standards. Copies of the first three sets of standards are included in the *Appendix* along with instructions on how to obtain the most recent editions of each.

Additional requirements may be included in state and/or local regulations and other organizations involved in long-term care. The *Appendix* includes a list of long-term care organizations from which more information can be obtained.

## PUTTING THE PACKAGE TOGETHER (Chapters 5 & 6)

If you are familiar with long-term care, you may begin planning and implementing service (Chapters 5 and 6). The planning and implementation process is dynamic. Whether you are serving LTCFs for the first time or have many years of experience, planning begins with evaluation, and evaluation continues throughout implementation and provision of service.

If you already serve a facility, evaluation means assessing the status of pharmaceutical service in the facility and judging where changes are needed. Change may come about because of growth of the facility or changes in the patient population. It may be due to regulatory or legal requirements, availability of new technologies, or external economic factors. Whatever the reason for changing methods of service, implementing new services, or revising compensation arrangements, change always requires planning.

If you have not previously served a LTCF, the evaluation process should include a self-evaluation of the services you desire and are able to provide and evaluation of the specific facility's needs for service. During planning, you should determine what services will be offered and to whom, what compensation will be expected, and how services will be promoted.

Once you have secured an agreement with a facility to provide service, you may begin implementation with a written contract that specifies the services to be provided, compensation arrangement, and other terms. You should prepare a manual containing the pharmaceutical service's policies and procedures in cooperation with other facility staff to further stipulate the services and how they will be performed. You should document the time spent providing service and monitor and evaluate the effectiveness of service continuously. The results of the evaluation should indicate when changes are needed.

The activities that occur in the planning and implementation phases have each been broken down into several steps in Chapters 5 and 6 to facilitate discussion of each phase.

During the planning phase, you will ask yourself what services will I provide; what are the needs of long-term care facilities; what services can I provide; and what course of action should I follow? During implementation, you may ask what will the contract contain; what will the policy and procedure manual contain; and how will I control and evaluate services?

As with any introductory text, this book leaves to the reader further investigation of many contemporary issues in LTCF practice. The references at the end of each chapter explore these issues in more detail.

What this book does is provide a stepwise foundation for the pharmacist interested in rewarding involvement in long-term care. With that foundation, the pharmacist's professional knowledge and management expertise should stand him or her in good stead.

1. McLeod, D. C. and F. M. Eckel, *J. Am. Pharm. Assn.*, NS9, 62(1969).

# Chapter 1:
# THE LONG-TERM CARE FACILITY

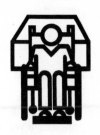

A long-term care facility (LTCF) is a facility or unit that is planned, staffed, and equipped to care for individuals who do not require acute hospital care but who are in need of nursing care and related health and social services. These services are prescribed by or performed under the supervision of persons licensed to provide such services or care in accordance with the laws of the state in which the facility is located. The primary aims and goals of a long-term care facility, as expressed in the philosophy of one long-term care association, are to preserve the dignity and worth of every individual and to meet the total emotional, physical, social, and spiritual needs of the residents. These goals are accomplished by providing well-equipped facilities, adequately staffed with qualified personnel.

## LEVELS OF CARE

To understand better the nature of care provided in long-term care facilities, let's see how they fit into the overall health care delivery system. LTCFs offer a level of care that is between the acute care of the hospital and care of the chronically ill in the home or through home health agencies, as the following descriptions indicate.

### Spectrum of Health Care Delivery[1]

**Intensive Care.** Intensive care/coronary care units (ICU/CCU) serve a lifesaving function, a level of care for those so seriously ill or injured that they need minute-by-minute monitoring. Typically, patients need this level of care only for short periods.

**Acute Care.** Acute care is that function traditionally performed by community hospitals. It is represented by a core of medical, surgical, pediatric, and obstetric inpatient beds, facilities, and services within the hospital for those who require it.

**Long-Term Care.** Long-term care services meet the needs of those patients whose requirements are such that they do not need to enter or remain in an acute care bed, but who still must have some nursing and medical treatment. Very often, long-term care also provides many rehabilitation services. Long-term care facilities are extensions (both before and after) of hospital care and are a level between the acute care hospital and home care. Long-term care is defined by Congress as health and/or personal care services required by persons who are chronically ill, aged, disabled, or retarded, in an institution, or at home, on a long-term basis. The term is often used more narrowly to refer only to long-term institutional care such as that provided in nursing homes, homes for the retarded, and mental hospitals.[2]

**Home Care.** Home care is an element of patient care that provides medical, nursing, social, rehabilitative, and related services on an intermittent basis in the home. Home care, which can also be provided on a long-term basis, is an alternative to institutionalization for the patient whose requirements can be met in the home.

**Outpatient Care.** Outpatient care is a level of care for patients who require diagnostic and therapeutic services not conveniently provided in the home. Outpatient services ordinarily are sufficient to meet the needs of most people. Group practice physicians' clinics, satellite health clinics, community pharmacies, and emergency rooms are basic outpatient care components. These facilities are very often the patient's point of entry into the health care system.

**Self-Care.** Through preventive health methods and educational processes, self-care helps people to manage their own health needs.

## Levels of Long-Term Care

The care provided in LTCFs is further subdivided into several levels. LTCFs are classified according to the level of care they provide in laws, regulations, and standards. In general, the level of care provided by the facility tells the public what services it should expect and the facility what services it must provide. Reimbursement to the facility is often based on the level of care. The definitions of LTCFs and levels of care vary from state-to-state. In an analysis of state laws, Aspen Systems Corporation found that the levels of care defined could be broken down into four categories: high, medium, minimum, and supervisory.[3] Classification of levels of care into one of these four categories may assist in comparing the requirements for service and compensation.

**High Level Category.** The institution has close relations with a staff of physicians who are readily available. Registered nurses are on duty 24 hours-a-day and medical and allied services of a high order are available.

**Medium Level Category.** A physician will be on call, and registered nurses are on duty 24 hours-a-day or licensed practical or vocational nurses are on duty under the supervision of a registered nurse. Prescribed medications may be administered and special diets provided.

**Minimum Level Category.** Assistance at meals and dressing along with supportive nursing care is available under the supervision of a licensed practical nurse.

**Supervisory Level Category.** Generally food, shelter, and laundry services are provided. The residents are primarily able to care for their own personal needs.

A facility may offer only one level of care or may offer different levels of care in separate sections of the facility. State licensure laws and federal regulations that contain definitions of levels of care include more detailed descriptions of the amount of staff required and the care to be provided. In addition, the patients in a facility offering a lower level of care may not be as ill as patients in a high level care facility, and therefore, may require fewer drugs and a different level of pharmaceutical service.

Examples of three levels of care defined by federal regulations are Skilled Nursing Facilities (SNFs), Intermediate Care Facilities (ICFs), and Intermediate Care Facilities in Institutions for the Mentally Retarded (ICF/MRs). These levels are set forth in the Medicare and Medicaid Conditions for Participation.

SNFs provide patients with continuous nursing service on a 24-hour basis. Registered nurses, licensed practical nurses, and nurses aides provide services prescribed by the patient's physician. Emphasis is on medical nursing care plus restorative, physical, and occupational therapy.

ICFs provide regular medical, nursing, and social services in addition to room and board for persons not capable of fully independent living. Intermediate Care Facilities in institutions for the mentally retarded offer the same services as other ICFs, as well as hygiene and rehabilitation services to train the residents to the fullest extent possible.

The National Center for Health Statistics (NCHS) also defines levels of care for its National Nursing Home Survey. Data collected in this survey are important in federal and state policy directions for long-term care. They indicate the number of patients, number of facilities, prevalence of disease states, average charges for care, and other valuable statistics on long-term care patients and facilities. The two levels defined by NCHS are nursing care home and personal care home.

The nursing care home provides skilled nursing care to at least 50% of its residents. The personal care home may provide some nursing care to less than 50% of its residents. Personal care includes assistance with bathing, dressing, walking, and eating.

The Joint Commission on the Accreditation of Hospitals (JCAH) is a private organization that defines two levels of care for its standards setting activities. They are the long-term health care facility and the resident care facility.

A long-term health care facility is a facility for inpatient care other than a hospital, with an organized medical staff, medical staff equivalent, or medical director, and with continuous nursing service under a professional nurse's direction. It is designed to provide, in addition to the medical care dictated by diagnoses, comprehensive preventive, rehabilitative, social, spiritual, and emotional inpatient care to individuals requiring long-term health care and to convalescent patients who have medical conditions with varying needs.

A resident care facility is a facility providing safe, hygienic living arrangements for residents. Regular and emergency health services are available when needed, and appropriate supportive services, including preventive, rehabilitative, social, spiritual, and emotional, are provided regularly.

These definitions demonstrate the variations found in descriptions of levels of care in long-term care facilities.

In Table 1-1, four categories developed by Aspen Systems are compared to the levels described in the different definitions.

Table 1-1

## LEVELS OF CARE

| Aspen Levels | Medicare & Medicaid | Joint Commission on the Accreditation of Hospitals | National Nursing Home Survey |
|---|---|---|---|
| High | Skilled Nursing Facility (SNF) | Long-Term Health Care Facility | Nursing Care Home |
| Medium | SNF, Intermediate Care Facility (ICF) & ICF in Institutions for the Mentally Retarded (ICF/MR) | Long-Term Health Care Facility | Nursing Care Home & Personal Care Home |
| Minimum | ICF & ICF/MR | Resident Care Facility | Personal Care Home |
| Supervisory | — | Resident Care Facility | Personal Care Home |

# OUTSIDE THE LTCF

The LTCF does not exist in a vacuum. It is within a complex system of community, governmental, and professional influences. As illustrated in Fig. 1-1, the objective of the LTCF is to convert ill patients, trained employees, and appropriate equipment and supplies into cared-for patients, satisfied employees, and improved community.

Outside the facility the patient is involved with relatives, friends, and third-party payers. The employees are involved with professional organizations and/or unions and governmental regulations. The facility as a whole is affected by laws and regulations, accreditation, and the community through planning agencies, fund raising, and publicity in the media. This complex array of external influences has caused many LTCFs to seek community awareness of and involvement in their services.

## State and Local Laws and Regulations

Just as each state licenses pharmacists and pharmacies, each also licenses LTCFs, the administrators, and many of the professional staff who practice within the facility. Through licensure laws, states may dictate staffing patterns, including the type of staff, ratio of staff to patients, and hours of coverage by certain professional staff. In some states, the licensure laws also include provisions requiring the facility to meet specific fire, safety, and hygiene regulations.

Facilities must also comply with local laws and ordinances. Among these are building construction codes, fire and safety codes, sanitary codes, zoning laws, and any law or ordinance affecting the health of the inhabitants of the county, city, town, or village.

Some state laws and regulations contain specific requirements for the pharmaceutical service which must be provided to a facility offering a given level of care. In some cases, the state pharmacy practice act includes requirements for pharmaceutical service in institutional settings.

Copies of the appropriate laws and regulations may be obtained from the state board of pharmacy, state department of health and/or welfare (or their equivalent), and state pharmaceutical association.

## Figure 1-1 — Outside of the Long-Term Care Facility

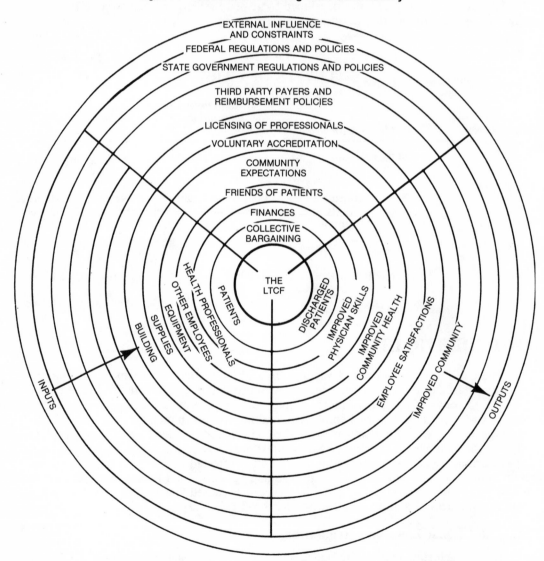

(Adapted with permission from *Management of Hospitals*, R. Schulz and A. C. Johnson, McGraw-Hill, New York, N.Y., 1976, p. 35.)

## Federal Regulations

For the most part, the federal regulations which affect LTCFs involve federal programs which provide money for them. For example, the Federal Housing Administration (FHA), which provides funds for the construction of new buildings, has a definition for "nursing homes" to which LTCFs receiving FHA funds must conform. LTCFs must also comply with federal regulations concerning minimum wage and equal opportunity employment. There are federal regulations concerning life and safety and accessibility to handicapped persons which apply to LTCFs.

## Medicare and Medicaid

The regulations which have had the greatest impact on pharmaceutical service are the Medicare and Medicaid Conditions for Participation. The Medicare and Medicaid regulations define two levels of care, described on page 2, for purposes of participation: the Skilled Nursing Facility (SNF) and the Intermediate Care Facility (ICF).

Medicare is financed entirely by federal funds. SNF services are covered for persons over 65 and others eligible to enroll for Part A of Medicare coverage. Drugs and biologicals supplied to beneficiaries in SNFs are covered by Medicare. The LTCF administration bills Medicare through a fiscal intermediary for all covered services on behalf of the providers. The pharmacist collects reimbursement for pharmaceutical services to Medicare patients from the facility. Approximately 1% of all long-term care facility patients are covered by Medicare.

The Medicaid program is financed by state and federal funds. It is designed to provide medical care to the medically and categorically needy. Both SNF and ICF services are covered by Medicaid. Drugs and biologicals provided to Medicaid beneficiaries in SNFs, ICFs, and as outpatients are covered. In most states, the pharmacist is reimbursed directly by Medicaid for drugs and related dispensing services. The pharmacist is compensated by the facility for nondispensing services; the facility then bills the state Medicaid agency.

Approximately 50% of all long-term care facility patients are covered by Medicaid.

The Medicare and Medicaid Conditions for Participation are contained in the article on the "Intent of the Regulations" by Samuel W. Kidder (see *Appendix*). The *Appendix* also contains instructions on how to obtain the most recent copy of the *Code of Federal Regulations* that lists the Conditions for Participation.

## Voluntary Standards

In addition to meeting the standards of care required by law, some LTCFs choose to seek voluntary accreditation by an independent standard setting agency.

The Accreditation Council for Long Term Care Facilities of the Joint Commission on Accreditation of Hospitals (JCAH) is an organization that seeks to recognize public facilities providing a high quality of care through a program of voluntary accreditation. JCAH awards accreditation based on the results of a survey of the facility. Surveys are conducted on invitation by those facilities interested in attaining the Council's recognition. Accreditation means that the facility has chosen to operate on the basis of standards developed by JCAH. While recognition is the principal outcome of accreditation, this process is considered more and more by government agencies and other third-party purchasers of care as the basis for certification to participate in their programs (often called "deemed status" from Section 1865 of the Social Security Act).

JCAH defines two levels of care, described on page 3, for the purposes of accreditation: the long-term health care facility and the resident care facility.

These two broad categories cover the various types of long-term care designated by governmental agencies for licensure, certification, and/or reimbursement purposes, including skilled nursing care and intermediate care. Determination of the category for accreditation purposes is made at the time of the survey, based on the primary role of the facility. If identifiable roles in both major areas can be determined, accreditation is considered in both categories (see Table 1-2 for definitions).

The *Appendix* contains information on how to obtain the most recent edition of the standards and a copy of the standards for Pharmaceutical Service in LTCFs. Information on how to obtain statements and policies adopted by several pharmaceutical organizations and LTCF organizations is also included in the *Appendix*. Some statements contained in these documents reflect the content of the regulations. However, in many cases, the standards suggested go beyond regulatory standards.

Table 1-2

## COMMONLY USED TERMS THAT REFER TO GOVERNMENTAL AND VOLUNTARY AUTHORITY OVER LTCFs

| | |
|---|---|
| **Licensure** | Required of all LTCFs |
| | Performed by state government agency according to state laws and regulations |
| **Certification** | Required for participation in Medicare and Medicaid |
| | Performed by state governmental agency according to Federal regulations and guidelines in addition to state regulations |
| **Accreditation** | Voluntary |
| | Performed by accrediting agency at invitation of LTCF |

# INSIDE THE LTCF

The influences inside the LTCF may be considered characteristics unique to a particular facility. They are divided into four categories: physical, ownership, patient, and staff. A few components of each category are discussed.

## Physical Characteristics

Physical characteristics of the facility include its location, size, age, design, and construction. The location of the building in relation to the pharmacy is particularly important if drugs are to be provided by an off-premises pharmacy, since the drugs must be delivered from the pharmacy to the LTCF. Building maintenance and design are important because the facility must have adequate drug storage areas and space for inservice training. The receiving areas, nursing stations, and general appearance of the building should be clean and well-kept. If the facility has an on-premises pharmacy, the space for the pharmacy must be large enough for all dispensing activities and should be readily accessible.

## Ownership Characteristics

LTCFs may be privately or publicly owned. They may be profit or nonprofit operations. Most LTCFs are proprietary (private, for profit) organizations.

The proprietary facilities may be owned by a single proprietor, a partnership, or corporation. They may be connected to a corporation by a franchise arrangement which includes an agreement to purchase certain goods and services and an entitlement to specific rights and duties. There are also chains of LTCFs owned by a single corporation.

Nonprofit LTCFs are owned and operated by nonprofit organizations, such as fraternal and religious orders, governmental units, or nonprofit hospitals.

The organizational entity determines the legal responsibilities and liabilities and affects the decisions of those operating the facility.

# Patient Characteristics

The characteristics of the patients and the number of patients are important to consider in providing pharmaceutical service. As mentioned previously, patients in a facility providing only a supervisory level of care are generally not as ill as those in a higher level care facility. They may require fewer drugs and less comprehensive service, or at least a different type of service than more seriously ill patients.

The number of beds, number of patients, and the fluctuation in occupancy rate are also critical. There may be seasonal fluctuations in occupancy. In addition, the patient mix affects the types of drugs ordered and the duration of treatment. Some facilities specialize in care of patients with diseases in a specific category, while others have a mixture of patients with wide variations in their drug needs.

These variables influence both dispensing and nondispensing services. The number and mix of patients affect the amount of drugs to be provided, frequency of delivery, and the time required to provide all pharmaceutical service. Fluctuation in occupancy and duration of treatment affect the cost of providing service, because there is a cost associated with each "admission to" and "discharge from" the drug distribution system. Also, a frequently changing patient population and frequently changing drug regimens increase the time required to perform patient drug therapy monitoring.

Statistics from the 1973-74 National Nursing Home Survey show that:

- Over 80% of the residents of LTCFs entered because of physical reasons, such as illness or need for treatment.
- Over one-half were admitted from another health facility, such as a hospital or another LTCF.
- Approximately 38% were admitted from a private residence.
- The median length of stay for all residents in the survey was 1.5 years.
- The average percent occupancy for all homes surveyed was 86.5% and the average rate of turnover was 0.9 admissions per bed per year.

These figures imply that long-term care facilities typically have very stable patient populations. Results of a survey conducted by the Department of Health, Education, and Welfare as part of the Long Term Care Facility Improvement Campaign indicated that the average number of prescriptions per patient in skilled nursing facilities is 6.1. The range in number of prescriptions ordered per patient was 0 to 23. The most frequently prescribed drug class was cathartics (prescribed to 58.1% of patients). Analgesics and tranquilizers were second and third (prescribed to 51.3% and 46.9% of patients, respectively.)[4]

# Staff Characteristics

The interrelationships among the staff and between the staff and the residents may have a greater impact on the day-to-day activities than any of the other charcteristics discussed. The policies and procedures established for all aspects of patient care direct these interrelationships. The functioning of the long-term care facility may be viewed as a system with all activity ultimately affecting the patients. Figure 1-2 illustrates one view of the internal organization with the patient at the center of all activity. Although the system is divided into Patient Care Programs, Support and Coordination, and the Medical Program, there is actually overlap in these activities daily. Because the pharmacist and the services which he or she provides are only a part of this activity, the pharmacist should understand the formal organizational structure and be sensitive to interpersonal and interprofessional relations.

Within the formal organizational structure, the pharmacist is responsible to the administrator for his or her actions. The administrator is the executive officer in charge who is responsible to the owner or governing board. As a licensed professional, the administrator has the daily legal responsibility for the facility's operation. The governing board or owner has ultimate legal responsibility for the administration. In some cases, the administrator is also the owner. Otherwise, the governing board assigns specific duties and responsibilities to the administrator. Figure 1-3 illustrates the formal internal structure.

The pharmacist also has a formally defined interaction with the director of nursing, the medical director, and the facility's physicians through participation on committees.

While the formal organizational structure provides the framework for staff interactions, personalities and other characteristics of the staff are most significant. The ideas and actions of the administrator and the director of nursing have a direct impact on all services. It is essential that the pharmacist establish good communication with these two individuals.

The number of physicians and their prescribing habits affect pharmaceutical service. If some physicians do not comply with the facility's policies and procedures concerning prescribing practices, effective informal lines of communication between the pharmacist and physicians may contribute greatly to resolving problems.

## Figure 1-2 — Inside of the Long-Term Care Facility

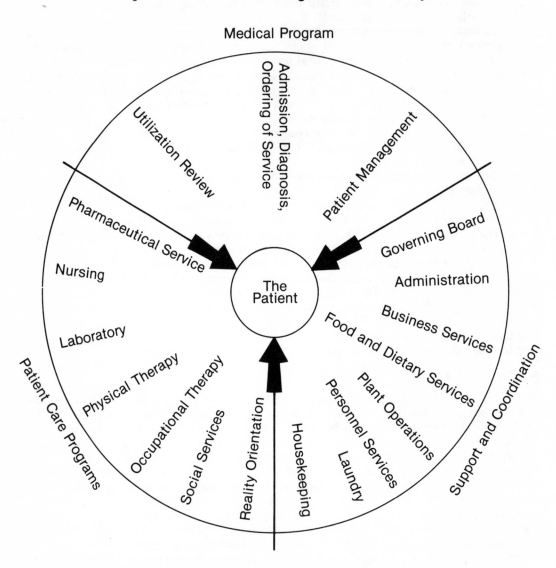

The pharmacist's informal communications are not limited to the administrator and nursing and medical staff. Other professionals serving the facility often include social workers, occupational therapists, physical therapists, dieticians, physician assistants, and possibly other pharmacists. Other personnel include nurses aides, housekeeping staff, and dietary workers. All personnel working in or serving a facility may interact at one time or another. The pharmacist should understand the responsibilities of various personnel and strive to achieve maximum cooperation with them.

**Figure 1-3 — Organization Chart for a Long-Term Care Facility**

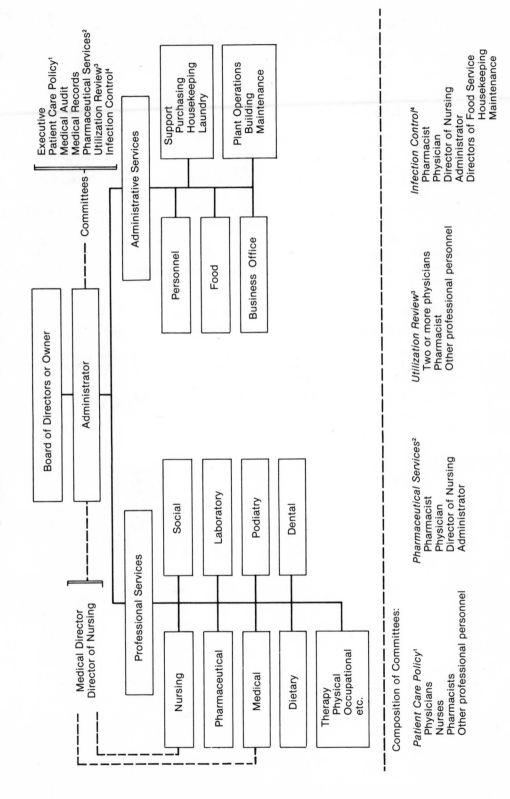

Committees

Executive
Patient Care Policy[1]
Medical Audit
Medical Records
Pharmaceutical Services[2]
Utilization Review[3]
Infection Control[4]

Board of Directors or Owner

Administrator

Medical Director
Director of Nursing

Professional Services

Administrative Services

Nursing
Social
Pharmaceutical
Laboratory
Medical
Podiatry
Dietary
Dental
Therapy
Physical
Occupational
etc.

Personnel
Food
Business Office

Support
Purchasing
Housekeeping
Laundry

Plant Operations
Building
Maintenance

Composition of Committees:

*Patient Care Policy[1]*
Physicians
Nurses
Pharmacists
Other professional personnel

*Pharmaceutical Services[2]*
Pharmacist
Physician
Director of Nursing
Administrator

*Utilization Review[3]*
Two or more physicians
Pharmacist
Other professional personnel

*Infection Control[4]*
Pharmacist
Physician
Director of Nursing
Administrator
Directors of Food Service
Housekeeping
Maintenance

9

1. Adapted from Baumgartner, R. P. *et al.*, "Home Health Agencies and the Pharmacist," *J. Amer. Pharm. Assn., NS14*, 355(1974).

2. *A Discursive Dictionary of Health Care*, Subcommittee on Health and the Environment, Committee on Interstate and Foreign Commerce, U.S. House of Representatives, Washington, D.C., February 1976.

3. *Nursing Home Law Manual*, Aspen Systems Corporation, Health Law Center, Germantown, Md., 1977.

4. *Physicians' Drug Prescribing Patterns in Skilled Nursing Facilities*, Long Term Care Facility Improvement Campaign, Monograph No. 2, U.S. Department of Health, Education and Welfare, Public Health Service, Office of Long Term Care, June 1976, Publication No. (OS) 76-50050.

## References for Further Reading

Abdellah, F. G., "The Future of Long-Term Care," *Bull. N.Y. Acad. Med., 54*, 261(1978).

*Data on Health Resources Utilization, Series 13*, "Statistics on the Utilization of Health Manpower and Facilities Providing Long-Term Care, Ambulatory Care, Hospital Care and Family Planning Services," Scientific and Technical Information Branch, National Center for Health Statistics, Public Health Service, Hyattsville, MD 20782.

Jones, E. W. *et al., Patient Classification for Long-Term Care: A User's Manual*, Department of Health, Education, and Welfare, Health Resources Administration, December 1973, Publication No. (HRA) 73-3107.

*Long-Term Care Facility Improvement Study, Introductory Report*, U.S. Department of Health, Education, and Welfare, Public Health Service, Office of Nursing Home Affairs, July 1975, Publication No. (OS) 76-50021.

McRae, D. C., "An Administrator Compares Long-Term Care and Acute Care Institutions," *J. Long-Term Care Admin., 6*, 17(Spring 1978).

*Nursing Home Costs—1972*, United States National Nursing Home Survey, August 1973—April 1974, U.S. Department of Health, Education, and Welfare, Public Health Service, November 1978, Publication No. (PHS) 79-1789.

*Nursing Home Law Manual*, Aspen Systems Corporation, Health Law Center, Germantown, Md., 1977.

*Physicians' Drug Prescribing Patterns in Skilled Nursing Facilities*, Long Term Care Facility Improvement Campaign, Monograph No. 2, U.S. Department of Health, Education, and Welfare, Public Health Service, Office of Long Term Care, June 1976, Publication No. (OS) 76-50050.

Schulz, R. and A. C. Johnson, *Management of Hospitals*, McGraw-Hill, New York, N.Y., 1976.

Smith, L. *et al.*, "Nurses' Perspective of Decision Making in Nursing Homes," *J. Long-Term Care Admin., 6*, 1(Winter 1978).

# Chapter 2:
# PHARMACEUTICAL SERVICES IN THE LTCF

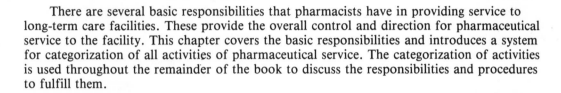

There are several basic responsibilities that pharmacists have in providing service to long-term care facilities. These provide the overall control and direction for pharmaceutical service to the facility. This chapter covers the basic responsibilities and introduces a system for categorization of all activities of pharmaceutical service. The categorization of activities is used throughout the remainder of the book to discuss the responsibilities and procedures to fulfill them.

## BASIC RESPONSIBILITIES

*Pharmacist's Responsibilities*

- Develops and implements systems for drug distribution, administration, and review in the long-term care facility
- Establishes and/or implements written policies and procedures for pharmaceutical service
- Reviews operations of the pharmaceutical service for compliance with local, state, and federal laws

Pharmaceutical services provided to a LTCF should create a system to ensure that the eight rights of drug therapy are followed: the right drug is administered to the right patient at the right time in the right amount using the right dosage form and the right route of administration to bring about a right, i.e., desired, response, and the right record is made of the drug administered and the response achieved. Drug therapy is an integral component of the care and treatment of most long-term care patients. A survey conducted by the Department of Health, Education, and Welfare revealed that an average of 6.1 drugs are prescribed for a skilled nursing facility patient. Some patients had prescription orders for as many as 23 drugs. Often these prescriptions were for conflicting or duplicative therapies. Therefore, LTCFs need pharmacists' services to monitor the appropriateness of therapy as well as provide an efficient and accurate means of distribution to and within the facility and administration to the patients. The pharmacist provides this service by creating a comprehensive medication system in cooperation with the administrator and other facility personnel.

The pharmacist establishes policies and procedures that delineate the total scope of pharmaceutical service to the facility. The policies and procedures should answer all questions regarding the ordering, receipt, administration, storage, disposition, and review of drugs in the facility; that is, they define control of the entire medication system (see also the section on policy and procedure manuals in Chapter 6).

Long-term care facilities may be served by pharmacists working in an on-premises or in one or more off-premises pharmacies. Freedom of choice provisions in federal and state laws and regulations allow more than one provider of dispensing services for patients in a given facility. However, if several pharmacies are providing services, they must all abide by the same policies and procedures.

The facility must make available adequate physical facilities and equipment to ensure compliance with the written pharmaceutical procedures and safe use of drugs. The responsibilities, functions, objectives, and terms of the pharmacists' services must be contained in a written agreement (see the section in Chapter 6 on contracts).

# THE MEDICATION SYSTEM

The medication system includes activities beginning with writing and processing the drug order, obtaining and storing the drugs, preparing and administering the individual doses, observing and recording the patient's response, and finally reviewing the need for continued therapy. The pharmacist's responsibilities regarding this medication system can be broken down into dispensing and nondispensing services. Dispensing services include activities associated with providing drug products. Pharmacies that provide drug products to LTCFs are sometimes called vendor, provider, or supplier pharmacies.

Nondispensing services include activities not directly connected to dispensing, such as drug regimen review, consultation with nurses and physicians, participation on committees, and provision of inservice training.

Figure 2-1 — **Pharmaceutical Service in the Long-Term Care Facility**

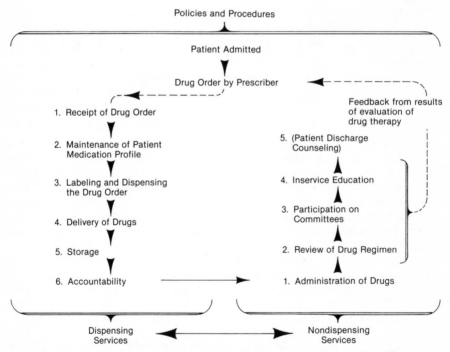

Figure 2-1 shows the sequence of activities that comprise the medication system, which begins with admission of the patient and initiation of the drug order by the prescriber and ends with patient discharge.

In reality, all of these activities are occurring simultaneously within a facility. However, if one patient is followed, the care of that patient can be thought of as a series of steps. Inherent in the steps is a constant review of the care of the patient in terms of drug therapy and pharmaceutical service (e.g., in maintenance of the patient medication profile, accountability of drugs, and review of the drug regimen). This analysis also categorizes all activities as either dispensing or nondispensing services.

# WHO PROVIDES SERVICES?

Depending on the circumstances, one pharmacist or a group working together may provide all of the pharmaceutical services required by the facility. In many cases, however, the pharmacist or group provides only a portion of the services with a separate and distinct individual or group providing the complement of services required by the facility. The set of services that the facility requires is determined by laws, regulations, standards, and its own unique needs. A pharmacist may be in the position to provide some or all of these services. The administrator is ultimately responsible for assuring that the facility is in compliance with legal requirements for services. Each pharmacist serving a facility should be aware of its total pharmaceutical service requirements, how his or her service fits into those requirements, and whether the facility is receiving all of the services it requires.

The following examples illustrate three approaches to serving long-term care facilities.

## Example 1

Pharmacist A owns a community pharmacy next door to Seabrook Nursing Home. Seabrook is a 150-bed facility in which most of the patients are skilled nursing patients. Seabrook's administrator asked pharmacist A to take over service to the facility because he had difficulty obtaining timely delivery service from the previous pharmacy, located 15 miles from the nursing home. Pharmacist A did not feel that he could serve the nursing home from his community practice, because of space limitations in his pharmacy. However, he did think that he could use some of his pharmacy staff and his own time to provide service to the facility from an on-premises pharmacy. Pharmacist A helped the administrator establish a licensed on-premises pharmacy and agreed to work as the pharmacist-in-charge. The laws in his state allow the pharmacy to be open only a few hours a day. From this on-premises pharmacy he and his staff provide the facility with all of its dispensing services. He chose to use a unit-dose drug distribution system. Pharmacist A also agreed to provide in-service training for facility staff and to participate on facility committees. The administrator hired Pharmacist B to conduct monthly drug regimen reviews for all patients and to provide the necessary communication and follow-up on the results of the reviews. Both pharmacists A and B inspect patient care areas regularly to assure that storage of drugs at nursing units complies with the facility's policies and procedures. The facility uses two separate providers to obtain its full complement of services.

## Example 2

Pharmacist C owns a community pharmacy and employs two full-time pharmacists. From this community pharmacy, they provide complete pharmaceutical service to several long-term care facilities, in addition to their community service. Each pharmacist spends several hours each week to provide all of the dispensing services to the facilities. They also share in the responsibilities of participation on the facilities' committees, providing inservice training, and conducting drug regimen reviews. Nonpharmacist personnel from the pharmacy deliver medication and perform administrative duties related to the nursing home service.

## Example 3

Five pharmacists are partners in a corporation that provides only the nondispensing services to long-term care facilities and small hospitals. Activities of the group include drug monitoring and counseling to both patients and medical staff, supportive services for community pharmacists, continuing education programs, and drug utilization review studies. The group provides all of the nondispensing services to a facility or only those services for which the facility wishes to contract. They serve long-term care facilities without dispensing a single drug.

The examples of the relationships between pharmacists and long-term care facilities and the selection of services they provide could go on; however, the services will still fall into the categories listed in Fig. 2-1. For cases in which the example pharmacists provide only a portion of the facility's complement of services, the remaining required services must be provided by other pharmacists.

Pharmaceutical services interface with activities of other members of the LTCF staff. The medication is ordered by a prescriber, usually administered by a nurse, according to policies and procedures approved by the facility's committees. The pharmacist provides and participates in inservice education with other staff members.

These activities and staff interactions are complex. The categorization of activities involved in pharmaceutical service is designed to provide a simple analysis of tasks to facilitate establishing policies and procedures, documentation of time spent providing services, and evaluation of service provided.

## References for Further Reading

*Accreditation Manual for Long-Term Care Facilities*, 1980 ed., Joint Commission on the Accreditation of Hospitals, 875 N. Michigan Avenue, Chicago, IL 60611, 1980.

Braverman, J., *Nursing Home Standards: A Tragic Dilemma in American Health Care*, American Pharmaceutical Association, Washington, D.C., 1970.

Cooper, J. W., "Drug Therapy in the Elderly: Is It All It Could Be?" *Am. Pharm., NS18*, 353(1978).

Gaeta, M. J. and R. J. Gaetano, *The Elderly: Their Health and the Drugs in Their Lives*, Kendall Hunt Publishing Co., 2460 Keeper Blvd., Dubuque, IA 52001, 1977.

"Guidelines for a Medical Director in a Long-Term Care Facility," Committee on Aging, Council on Medical Services, American Medical Association, Chicago, Ill., 1974.

Kalman, S. H. and J. F. Schlegel, "Introduction: Standards of Practice," *Am. Pharm., NS19*, 134(1979).

Kidder, S. W., "Skilled Nursing Facilities—A Clinical Opportunity for Pharmacists," *Am. J. Hosp. Pharm., 34*, 751(1977).

"Minimum Standards for Pharmacies in Institutions," *Am. J. Hosp. Pharm., 34*, 1356(1977).

*A National Study of the Practice of Pharmacy*, American Pharmaceutical Association and American Association of Colleges of Pharmacy, Washington, D.C., 1978.

*Nursing Home Care in the United States: Failure in Public Policy*, "Supporting Paper No. 2—Drugs in Nursing Homes: Misuse, High Costs and Kickbacks," Subcommittee on Long-Term Care, Select Committee on Aging, United States Senate, Washington, D.C., 1975.

*Pharmaceutical Services in the Long-Term Care Facility*, 7th ed., American Health Care Association, American Pharmaceutical Association, and American Society of Hospital Pharmacists, Washington, D.C., 1975.

Reichel, W. (ed.), *Clinical Aspects of Aging*, Williams and Wilkins, Baltimore, MD 21202, 1978.

"Statement on Hospital Drug Control Systems," *Am. J. Hosp. Pharm., 31*, 1196(1974).

*Title 42 CFR 405.1101-1137* Conditions for Participation for Skilled Nursing Facilities in Medicare and Medicaid, HEW, HCFA, 1979.

*Title 42 CFR 442.300-346* Standards for Intermediate Care Facilities other than Facilities for the Mentally Retarded for Medicaid, HEW, HCFA, 1979.

*Title 42 CFR 442.400-516* Standards for Intermediate Care Facilities for the Mentally Retarded for Medicaid, HEW, HCFA, 1979.

# Chapter 3:
# DISPENSING SERVICES

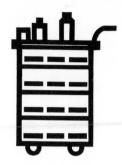

As indicated in Fig. 2-1, dispensing services are subdivided into receipt of the drug order, maintenance of patient medication profile, labeling and dispensing the drug order, delivery, storage, and accountability. The pharmacist's responsibilities for each function and procedures commonly used are given in this chapter.

## RECEIPT OF DRUG ORDER

*Pharmacist's Responsibilities*

- Verifies the prescription order for completeness and accuracy
- Verifies the prescription order for amount per dose, appropriate route, frequency, duration of therapy, and applicability of stop orders

### Procedures

The procedures for sending drug orders to the pharmacy should ensure that the original prescriber's order is transmitted accurately. The facility obtains patients' drug orders from the authorized prescriber through a written or oral order. Only a nurse, pharmacist, or physician may receive verbal orders. Verbal orders must be recorded and signed by the person receiving the order. They must be countersigned by the prescribing physician within 48 hours. The signed order is incorporated into the patient's health records.

The pharmacy may receive the original written order signed by the prescriber or a direct copy. Oral orders may be sent to the pharmacy by the prescriber or by facility staff acting as the prescriber's agent where permitted by state laws and regulations. When a new patient is admitted, the orders are often telephoned to the pharmacy by the facility; however, the pharmacy must receive a copy of the signed prescriber's order as soon as possible.

The pharmacist should preferrably dispense from the original written order or a direct copy thereof.

Drug orders typically contain the following information:
- Correct and complete name of patient
- Physician's name and telephone number
- Patient's billing status
- Patient's admission number, if appropriate
- Patient's allergy history
- Patient's admitting diagnosis
- Drugs ordered with quantity and directions for use
- Facility nursing station
- Name of nurse calling order, if appropriate

Each order should be reviewed for completeness and for any needed clarification. In some instances, a conversion of some of the text of the order to standard abbreviations that have been established for the facility through the pharmaceutical services committee may be necessary. For example, all dosages may be expressed in the metric system or certain generic drug names may be reduced to standard abbreviations.

The pharmaceutical services committee should establish some ground rules for the use of abbreviations in the writing of medication orders. Criteria should be established for expressing drug strengths and quantities to be administered. A list of commonly used abbreviations for drug names could be developed and posted at each nursing station. A metric system conversion table and a list of committee-approved abbreviations for order writing should be posted to reduce potential errors in drug administration.

## Physicians' Orders

Figure 3-1 is an example of a physician's order form. The physician writes the orders in the spaces on this sheet. The patient information legend at the end of the form is completed when the form is placed in the patient's health record. The facility must provide a copy of the physician's order to the pharmacy. A carbon or photocopy of this order form may be sent. Some pharmacies have copies of original orders transmitted daily by use of a telecopier.

The form in Fig. 3-2 can be used conveniently for a monthly recap of the patient's orders. The physician reviews and signs the recap under the last order, to authorize continuation.

## Stop Order Policy

An important step in the receipt of the medication order is to review the applicability of the facility's stop order policy. A stop order is an order to stop a treatment. The policy established by the pharmaceutical services committee outlines when a stop order should be used. The stop order may limit the length of time a treatment may be administered before contacting a physician for renewal. It may be for all drugs, a specific drug, a general drug category, class, or treatment type. The stop order should be used only when the prescriber does not limit the time or number of doses to be administered. For example, some facilities impose stop orders of 2 weeks on all orders of antibiotics. If the prescriber does not specify the duration of therapy or the number of doses to be administered, the facility staff must contact him or her near the end of the 2-week period to obtain authorization to continue the therapy beyond the 2-week stop order limit. Ideally, a stop order should be required rarely; however, to expect that all orders will be written in such complete detail that a stop order policy will not be needed is unrealistic.

**Figure 3-1**

PHYSICIAN'S ORDERS AND SIGNATURE FORM

| FACILITY | NUMBER |

| PROBLEM NUMBER | ORDERS & SIGNATURE | DATE & TIME |

GENERIC EQUIVALENT DRUG MAY BE DISPENSED UNLESS CHECKED HERE ☐

| LAST NAME | FIRST NAME | INIT. | ATTENDING PHYSICIAN | ROOM NO. | PATIENT NUMBER |

**CHART COPY**

**Figure 3-2**

# PHYSICIANS PLEASE NOTE

TO VALIDATE RECAP PHYSICIANS ORDER SHEET, PHYSICIAN SHOULD DATE AND SIGN UNDER LAST ORDER, EVERY 30 DAYS

| R NUMBER | DATE ORIGINATED | * | PHYSICIANS ORDERS ASTERISK INDICATES NEW ORDER THIS MONTH |
|---|---|---|---|
| | | | |

PHYSICIAN NAME · PHONE NO. · ALTERNATE · ALT. PHONE NO.

ALLERGIES

DIAGNOSIS

RESTORATIVE POTENTIAL

PATIENT'S NAME · PATIENT NO. · ROOM NO. · ADMIT DATE · AGE · SEX · HEIGHT · WEIGHT · MO/YR · PAGE NO.

# MAINTENANCE OF PATIENT MEDICATION PROFILE

*Pharmacist's Responsibilities*

- Maintains a record file of current prescription orders and renewal data
- Maintains a record file of pertinent patient information
- Checks patient records for pertinent patient information before dispensing prescription medication
- Interviews the patient or his/her representative for entry into the patient record, patient profile, or health record, when appropriate
- Updates the patient's history in the patient's medication record from information obtained from the patient's records or recurring patient interviews

## Procedures

Contemporary pharmacy practice and services require the use of medication profiles to assist the pharmacist in monitoring the effectiveness of drug therapy. A medication profile affords the pharmacist an opportunity to monitor the patient's drug therapy on a "before-the-fact" basis in addition to reviewing the patient's drug regimen monthly in the facility "after-the-fact" of drug administration. It is almost inconceivable that a pharmacist can perform adequately without the use of a medication profile, either in a manual or a computerized system, regardless of the drug distribution system in use.

The format of the profile should be such that the pharmacist can readily review all current PRN and routine drugs the patient is receiving, the frequency of dispensing, basic patient data such as age, weight, sex, allergy, diagnosis, physician(s), address or facility location, patient billing type, and any other information or data that a particular pharmacist's practice may require.

In some states, a properly designed profile can also be used as the complete prescription record by including the prescription number, directions, and other appropriate information to meet the state board of pharmacy requirements for a prescription record. Use of a profile as the prescription record eliminates the necessity of maintaining two separate filing systems for the patient's medication history.

Figure 3-3 is an example of a patient profile on which a record of renewals of drug orders may be retained for 12 months. The back of the profile form contains space for pharmacist's notes. The notes might include such items as consultations between the pharmacist and prescribers, consultations with nursing personnel, information on drug therapy, etc. This particular profile card is designed to be maintained in the pharmacy with copies provided to the facility.

The pharmacist is responsible for the accuracy of the patient profile/prescription record. Initial patient information and subsequent changes to non-technical patient information may be entered by nonlicensed pharmacy personnel. All other entries are made by the pharmacist.

Sources of information for the patient medication profile are drug orders, the attending nurses, other pharmacists, the patient and written information from the facility's records, such as the admission form, night nurse report, patient change of status form, and copies of physician's orders.

## Obtaining Patient Data

Patient data may be obtained in several ways. Most facilities have an admission form that contains some of the basic data described in the discussion of patient profiles. Nursing and office personnel who contact the facility or institution from which the patient is being transferred and/or the family obtain most of the necessary information.

Nursing personnel call the transferring institution to confirm the admission and timing and to ensure that transfer of records will be complete, including appropriate diagnosis for admission to the facility. They inquire as to the specific condition of the patient and the nursing procedures that will be carried out in the convalescent setting. The director of nurs-

Figure 3-3

| Patient | | Billing Status | | Physician | | Diagnosis |
|---|---|---|---|---|---|---|
| Pat. No. | | I. D. No. | | Phys. Phone | | |
| Facility | | Phys. Address | | | | |
| Address | | DEA No. | | Allergies/Idiosyncrasies | | |
| City | | Lic. No. | | | | |
| Admission Date | | Prod. Sel. | | | | |
| Date of Birth | | Disch. Date | NF | | | |
| S. S. No. | | I. D.s | ↑ | | | |

| MEDICATION | Rx NUMBER | DIRECTIONS | QTY. | Fee Code | JAN | FEB | MAR | APR | MAY | JUN | JUL | AUG | SEP | OCT | NOV | DEC |
|---|---|---|---|---|---|---|---|---|---|---|---|---|---|---|---|---|
| | | | | | | | | | | | | | | | | |
| | | | | | | | | | | | | | | | | |
| | | | | | | | | | | | | | | | | |
| | | | | | | | | | | | | | | | | |
| | | | | | | | | | | | | | | | | |
| | | | | | | | | | | | | | | | | |
| | | | | | | | | | | | | | | | | |
| | | | | | | | | | | | | | | | | |

ing may have to make a preliminary choice of the section of the facility in which to place the patient.

Office personnel contact the appropriate personnel in the transferring institution and business office to ascertain the sources of reimbursement that are paying for the long-term care facility stay; who is responsible for the patient's affairs and pays the bills; what the payment record has been where private funds are involved; and any credit data which the hospital or other facility will release. Office personnel also contact the patient's responsible family member or other legally responsible person to obtain any preadmission information, including credit information, and to answer any questions regarding facility policies and the pending admission.

The patient's physician should be contacted only by licensed nursing personnel or the administrator and occasionally, licensed therapists and pharmacists, when contact is required (a) to determine if the physician will visit the patient in the facility or if arrangements will be made to transport the patient to the physician's office; (b) to clarify diagnosis, orders for nursing or therapy procledures; (c) or for administration of medications. Personnel from the facility obtain the necessary authorization required prior to admitting the Medicaid or welfare patient. A typical admission form has three parts: the original top copy (Fig. 3-4) to be placed in the medical record, a form to be filled out if the patient dies, and a copy for the facility's master file of patient information.

In some cases the pharmacist may find that it is desirable to conduct an admission interview (Fig. 3-5) with the patient and/or the family. The pharmacist may use a form such as that illustrated in Fig. 3-6 to report the results of this interview to the physician(s) responsible for care of the patient.

# LABELING AND DISPENSING THE DRUG ORDER

*Pharmacist's Responsibilities*

- Establishes a drug distribution system for the facility
- Performs packaging and labeling functions to promote product stability
- Verifies prescription orders for physical and chemical compatibility
- Measures quantities needed to dispense the prescription
- Compounds the prescribed ingredients according to a prescription formula or instructions
- Reconstitutes lyophilized or powdered pharmaceuticals into dosage forms suitable for administration, when appropriate
- Selects appropriate labeling for prescription container and includes patient instructions
- Performs a final check of the finished product to ensure that each step has been accomplished accurately

The dispensed medication is channeled into the drug distribution and administration system. To develop and implement a system for drug distribution and administration, the pharmacist may also do the following:

- Initiate a formulary system to meet the needs of patients and practitioners
- Establish drug quality specifications for drugs to be purchased
- Select the manufacturing source of drug products to be dispensed for a brand name prescription order in those cases where legally authorized
- Develop and maintain quality control records for drugs that are prepackaged, bulk compounded, sterile product formulated, etc.

Figure 3-4

# ADMISSION
# INFORMATION

| | |
|---|---|
| 1 | FACILITY NUMBER |
| | MEDICAL CHART |

| 2 | PATIENT'S LAST NAME | FIRST NAME | M. I. | PATIENT NUMBER | ADMISSION DATE & TIME |

| 3 | PATIENT'S ADDRESS — STREET, CITY, STATE, ZIP. |

| 4 | BIRTH DATE | AGE | BIRTH PLACE | SEX | RACE | CITIZENSHIP | RELIGION | MARITAL STATUS M S D W SEP | ROOM | BED |

| 5 | ATTENDING PHYSICIAN(S) | TELEPHONE NO. | ADDRESS | CITY | STATE | ZIP |
| | ADDITIONAL PHYSICIAN | TELEPHONE NO. | ADDRESS | CITY | STATE | ZIP |
| 6 | ALTERNATE PHYSICIAN | TELEPHONE NO. | ADDRESS | CITY | STATE | ZIP |
| 7 | ATTENDING DENTIST | TELEPHONE NO. | ADDRESS | CITY | STATE | ZIP |
| 8 | NEXT OF KIN — IN EMERGENCY | TELEPHONE NO. | ADDRESS | CITY | STATE | ZIP |
| 9 | NEXT OF KIN — IN EMERGENCY | TELEPHONE NO. | ADDRESS | CITY | STATE | ZIP |
| 10 | RESPONSIBLE PARTY (Conservator, etc.) | TELEPHONE NO. | ADDRESS | CITY | STATE | ZIP |

| 11 | ADMITTING DIAGNOSIS | MEDICARE NO. |

| 12 | ALLERGIES | MEDICAID / MEDICAL NO. |

| 13 | HOSPITAL ADMITTED FROM (Qualifying Hospital Stay) | DATE OF QUALIFYING STAY (Medicare) Admitted   Discharged |

| 14 | OTHER PRIOR HOSPITAL / SNF STAY INFORMATION 1. |

| 15 | 2. |

| 16 | USUAL OCCUPATION | FATHER'S NAME | MOTHER'S MAIDEN NAME | MILITARY SERVICE - DATES OF SERVICE (If available) |

## BILLING DATA

| 17 | BILL TO (name) | INITIAL PATIENT TYPE | CODE | SECONDARY PATIENT TYPE | CODE |
| 18 | BILL TO (address line 1) | PVT. CONTRACT RATE $ | CODE | ESTIMATED LIABILITY $ | |
| 19 | BILL TO (address line 2) | SOCIAL SECURITY NUMBER | | THIRD PARTY I. D. NUMBER | |
| 20 | BILL TO (address line 3) | WELFARE CASE WORKER | | | |

| 21 | MEDICAID ONLY | MEDI-CARE STATUS CODE | MEDI-CARE BENEFITS Exhausted Date | I.D. CARD REC'D ON ADMISSION yes    no | ATTENDING PHYSICIAN'S STATE LICENSE NUMBER | V. A. NUMBER | PRIOR PATIENT NUMBER |

*INSTRUCTIONS:*
1. Shaded information **must** be obtained upon admission.
2. Distribute Chart Copy to nursing on day of admission.

## DISCHARGE INFORMATION

| 22 | MORTUARY | TELEPHONE |

| 23 | DISCHARGE DIAGNOSIS (1.) |

| 24 | DISCHARGE DIAGNOSIS (2.) |

| 25 | DISPOSITION | ICDA CODE | DISCHARGE DATE |

| PATIENT NAME | ATTENDING PHYSICIAN | PATIENT NUMBER |

Figure 3-5 — **Survey**

Health Care
Facility _____

Patient's Name _____
Physician(s) _____

TO: The Patient or Your Family

## MEDICATION SURVEY

1. The purpose of this survey is to gather as much data as we possibly can concerning the medications which you have taken over the past several months. This information will be tabulated and communicated to your physician so that he or she will have available a complete picture of your medication history.

   All data furnished is solely hospital or nursing home property and will be treated with strict confidentiality. Please provide as much information as you can.

2. Please list the names and addresses of pharmacies or drug stores where you have had prescriptions filled in the last six months:

   NAME                                          ADDRESS

   _____
   _____
   _____
   _____

3. Please list the names of all doctors, dentists, podiatrists, or other persons who you have seen for health needs in the past six months.

   _____
   _____
   _____
   _____

4. Please list the medications, both prescription and non-prescription, that you have been taking over the last year. If you do not know the name of the medications, please list the prescription number and pharmacy where obtained, and give the best physical description of the drug (color, size, shape, etc.) If possible, please bring in all your current medications for identification. They will be returned to you after they have been identified.

   The following list may help you to remember some of the medications, drugs or patent medicines or "cures" you have taken. Please give as much information as possible. Thank you.

(Courtesy of James W. Cooper, Jr., Ph.D., University of Georgia, School of Pharmacy, Athens, Ga.)

Have you, in the last 6 months, taken or been advised to take any of the following for:

| | Symptoms | Drugs | How Long (days, weeks, months) |
|---|---|---|---|
| 4.1 | "Irregularity" "Constipation" | ____ Milk of Magnesia<br>____ Ex-Lax, Dulcolax<br>____ Mineral Oil, Haley's MO<br>____ Other _____ | _____<br>_____<br>_____<br>_____ |
| 4.2 | "Diarrhea" "Runny Stools" | ____ Kaopectate, Pepto-Bismol<br>____ Donnagel, Lactinex, Lomotil Paregoric | _____<br>_____ |
| 4.3 | "Upset Stomach" "Ulcer Medication" | ____ Alka-Seltzer, Bromo-Seltzer<br>____ Baking Soda<br>____ Tums, Rolaids<br>____ Celusil, Maalox, Mylanta<br>____ Other _____ | _____<br>_____<br>_____<br>_____<br>_____ |
| 4.4 | Aches and Pains "Headaches" "Arthritic and Rheumatic Pain" | ____ Aspirin, Anacin<br>____ Bufferin, BC Powders<br>____ Codeine, Darvon, Demerol<br>____ Decadron, Cortisone, Prednisone<br>____ Other _____ | _____<br>_____<br>_____<br>_____<br>_____ |
| 4.5 | Eye Preparations "Glaucoma" "Red, irritated eyes" | ____ Phospholine-Iodide<br>____ Humorsol, Isopto-Carpine<br>____ Visine, Pilocarpine<br>____ Other _____ | _____<br>_____<br>_____<br>_____ |
| 4.6 | Ear Preparations | ____ Auralgan<br>____ Other _____ | _____<br>_____ |
| 4.7 | Colds Hayfever Stuffy Nose | ____ Antihistamines<br>____ Aspirin, Tylenol<br>____ Neo-Synephrine<br>____ Cold Tablets, Contac<br>____ Cough Syrup, Nyquil<br>____ Other _____ | _____<br>_____<br>_____<br>_____<br>_____<br>_____ |
| 4.8 | Birth Control GYN "The Pill" | ____ Oral Contraceptives<br>____ Other _____ | _____<br>_____ |
| 4.9 | "Heart Medications" | ____ Digitalis<br>____ Nitroglycerin<br>____ Quinidine, Pronestyl<br>____ Other _____ | _____<br>_____<br>_____<br>_____ |
| 4.10 | "High Blood Pressure" "Water Pills" "Potassium" | ____ Diuril (Water Pill)<br>____ Reserpine, Ser-Ap-Es<br>____ Aldomet<br>____ Esimil<br>____ Catapres, Inderal<br>____ Kaochlor<br>____ Klorvess<br>____ Slow-K | _____<br>_____<br>_____<br>_____<br>_____<br>_____<br>_____<br>_____ |
| 4.11 | Asthma, Bronchitis Emphysema | ____ Tedral, Amesec, Bronkotabs<br>____ Prednisone<br>____ Isuprel Aerosol<br>____ Epinephrine Aerosol<br>____ Decadron, Cortisone<br>____ Other _____ | _____<br>_____<br>_____<br>_____<br>_____<br>_____ |
| 4.12 | "Nerve Pills" | ____ Librium, Thorazine<br>____ Valium, Mellaril<br>____ Meprobamate (Miltown, Equanil)<br>____ Other _____ | _____<br>_____<br>_____<br>_____ |
| 4.13 | Insomnia | ____ Sominex, Nytol, Dalmane<br>____ Seconal, Doriden, Quaalude<br>____ Nembutal, Noludar, Noctec<br>____ Chloral Hydrate<br>____ Other _____ | _____<br>_____<br>_____<br>_____<br>_____ |

| 4.14 | Antibiotics "Infections" | ____ Penicillin | _____ |
| | | ____ Tetracycline | _____ |
| | | ____ Erythromycin | _____ |
| | | ____ Sulfa | _____ |
| | | ____ Other _____ | _____ |
| 4.15 | Blood Clotting "Blood Thinners" "Anticoagulants" | ____ Coumadin | _____ |
| | | ____ Heparin | _____ |
| | | ____ Other _____ | _____ |
| 4.16 | "Blood Builders" Anemia Drugs | ____ Iron tablets, Geritol | _____ |
| | | ____ Fem-Iron | _____ |
| | | ____ Folic Acid | _____ |
| | | ____ $B_{12}$ Shots | _____ |
| | | ____ Vitamins | _____ |
| | | ____ Other _____ | _____ |
| 4.17 | Diabetes | ____ Insulin | _____ |
| | | ____ Orinase | _____ |
| | | ____ Diabinese | _____ |
| | | ____ Other _____ | _____ |
| 4.18 | Hemorrhoids | ____ Anusol | _____ |
| | | ____ Preparation H | _____ |
| | | ____ Medicone, Tucks | _____ |
| | | ____ Other _____ | _____ |
| 4.19 | Skin Conditions—dry Eczema, Psoriasis Athletes Foot, Corns Dandruff, Infections | ____ Neosporin | _____ |
| | | ____ Tegrin, Mazon | _____ |
| | | ____ Keri, Vioform | _____ |
| | | ____ Other _____ | _____ |
| 4.20 | Other Conditions | _____ | _____ |
| | | _____ | _____ |
| | | _____ | _____ |
| | | _____ | _____ |
| | | _____ | _____ |

5. Do you or have you ever had:

5.1  Any problems with drugs? ____ Yes ____ No (Please list)

_____

_____

_____

5.2  Any allergies to foods, drugs, pets, environment? ____ Yes ____ No

5.3  A family history of allergy? ____ Yes ____ No

5.4  A drug discontinued because of: rash, itching, nausea, vomiting?
____ Yes ____ No

5.5  Difficulty in swallowing tablets or capsules? ____ Yes ____ No

5.6  Or been told that you've had a reaction to a drug, shot, or medicine?
____ Yes ____ No

5.7  Have you been in a hospital in the last year? ____ Yes ____ No
If yes, which hospital? _____

6. Please return this form to your pharmacist as soon as possible.

**Figure 3-6**

# HEALTH CARE FACILITY
## Notice of Medication History

Physician's Name _____

Patient's Name _____ Room Number _____

Members of the Pharmacy Department staff have compiled a medication history via an interview with your patient.

1. Medications which your patient was taking upon admission to the facility are listed for your information below:

|  | COMPLIANCE | | | | |
| MEDICATION | Yes | Irreg. | No | Presc. No. | Pharmacy |
| --- | --- | --- | --- | --- | --- |
|  |  |  |  |  |  |
|  |  |  |  |  |  |
|  |  |  |  |  |  |
|  |  |  |  |  |  |
|  |  |  |  |  |  |

2. Verified sensitivities, allergies or adverse reactions:

   a. Drugs

   b. Food

   c. Environment

3. Pharmacist's Remarks: _____

_____

_____

_____

_____
                              (Pharmacist's Name)

(Courtesy of James W. Cooper, Jr., Ph.D., University of Georgia, School of Pharmacy, Athens, Ga.)

# Procedures

Accuracy of the prescription label and the medication is of paramount importance. Once the medication order has been validated, the physical process of dispensing takes place. The type of drug distribution system in use by the pharmacy for a particular facility will have specific procedures that must be followed to ensure accurate administration. The procedures will vary depending on the type of system and equipment involved.

## Drug Distribution Systems

Drug distribution systems vary in the type of packaging used and the number of total days of dosage units supplied to the facility. The packaging used includes traditional prescription containers (vials and bottles), plastic containers with dividers separating each dose, blister package cards, single unit dose blister packages, and liquid and ointment containers. The number of dosage units supplied may vary from a 24-hour supply to 1 month or 30 days, or occasionally a larger supply. The drug distribution systems most commonly used can be divided into two categories: traditional and unit dose. There are many variations within these categories, but the following discussion describes the distinguishing characteristics of each system.

**Traditional System.** In this system the prescription containers are the traditional vials for solid dosage forms and bottles for liquids. A 30-day or 1-month supply of chronic drugs is generally dispensed. Some state Medicaid programs require 100 units of certain drugs to be dispensed. Labeling on the traditional prescription container is similar to the labeling required for outpatient prescriptions. There may be some differences from outpatient labeling based on policies and procedures adopted by the facility or required by state laws and regulations, such as inclusion of lot numbers and expiration date. At the nursing unit, the prescription containers may be stored in permanently affixed drug cabinets or in specially designed carts with compartments large enough to hold these relatively bulky packages.

Because many doses of the drug are dispensed in each vial or bottle, the nurse administering the drug must pour the individual doses prior to administration. Trays with drug or souffle cups and drug schedule cards are used to hold the drugs until they are administered.

**Blister Cards and Plastic Divided Boxes.** The use of multidose packages in which each dosage unit is physically separated is a variation of the traditional system. Generally, a 30-day or 1-month supply is dispensed. Labeling in this modification of the traditional system is the same as on prescription vials or containers, as are the administration procedures. Use of these systems requires special packaging equipment and specially designed carts for storage at the nursing units.

The main difference between these systems and the strictly traditional system is that the number of doses remaining can be counted easily without disturbing the integrity of the package. In addition, each package compartment is numbered. Use of the dose from the numbered compartment that corresponds to the date of administration decreases the likelihood of dosing errors present in the traditional system. Doses may be divided by administration time, also decreasing or identifying dosing errors. The procedure of pouring by the nurse is eliminated and the drug is identified to the point of administration. This system is also useful for maintaining accountability of controlled substances.

**Unit Dose.** A single definition of a unit dose drug distribution system in the long-term care facility has not been generally accepted by pharmacists practicing in long-term care. In a true unit dose distribution system, as defined in hospitals, all drugs (solids, liquids, and ointments) are dispensed in single unit packages. In most unit dose distribution systems in long-term care facilities, only solid oral dosage forms are supplied in single unit packages. The amount supplied varies from a 1-day (24-hours) to 7-day supply. The drugs are supplied and stored at the nursing unit in carts containing individual patient containers, bins, compartments, or drawers and doses are subdivided by administration time. Labeling requirements for each package have been described in several statements.

Because the individual doses are divided according to time of administration in the storage containers and each dose is packaged individually, the nurse administering the drugs need not pour the drugs before administration. This procedure, combined with the fact that each dose is identified up to the time of administration, offers the smallest possibility of dosing errors of the three systems described.

In the unit dose systems used in most long-term care facilities, only solid oral dosage forms are supplied in single unit packages. Medications packaged in traditional packages must be treated in the same manner as in a traditional system. Use of a mixture of systems may decrease the effectiveness of some of the advantages cited for a unit dose system.

**Floor Stock.** The floor stock system was at one time "the system" of drug distribution in hospitals. In this system, a bulk supply of the drug is kept at the nursing unit. This system is not used in long-term care facilities for legend drugs. However, because of the reimbursement mechanisms in some states, the floor stock system is currently used for nonlegend (OTC) drugs in combination with the three systems described. The incentive for use of nonlegend floor stock drugs is economic, but the practice should be discouraged. The floor stock system removes control of part of the medication system from the pharmacist and complicates the factors used to assess patients' drug therapy. For nursing home patients receiving complex multiple therapy, inappropriate use of nonlegend drugs represents a threat of disruption of the entire course of therapy.

**Record Keeping.** Appropriate records are an integral component of all drug distribution systems. Maintenance of patient medication profiles and drug administration records to optimize drug control are necessary,regardless of the distribution system used; these are described elsewhere in this chapter.

Table 3-1 summarizes the major advantages and disadvantages of each distribution system. The final choice is usually based on convenience, economy, and the system which affords the best control over drug use in the facility.

**Table 3-1**

## Summary of Advantages and Disadvantages of
## Three Systems of Drug Distribution

| | *Advantages* | *Disadvantages* |
|---|---|---|
| Traditional | Less frequent dispensing of individual prescriptions. Fits into community practice. No special equipment. Less personnel to dispense. Less cost. | Less control and accountability. Greatest possibility for dosing errors. More nursing time. Bulky storage. |
| Blister Card | Less frequent dispensing. Better control than traditional. Less chance of dosing errors. Less nursing time. | Requires special equipment. May require additional personnel for dispensing. Bulky storage. Greater cost. Cumbersome when associated with frequent alterations of drug therapy. |
| Unit Dose | Best control. Least chance of dosing errors. Least waste of unused medications. Less nursing time. | Requires special equipment. More pharmacist time. May not be reimbursable. Greater cost. May require additional personnel for dispensing. |

Figure 3-7
**UNIT DOSE WORK SHEET**

MONTH _____

| DATES | MEDICATIONS | CODE | QUANTITY DISPENSED 1 | 2 | 3 | 4 | 5 | 6 | 7 | 8 | 9 | 10 | 11 | 12 | 13 | 14 | 15 | 16 | TD |
|---|---|---|---|---|---|---|---|---|---|---|---|---|---|---|---|---|---|---|---|
| START | ℞ No. | | 17 | 18 | 19 | 20 | 21 | 22 | 23 | 24 | 25 | 26 | 27 | 28 | 29 | 30 | 31 | 16 | |
| RENEW | | | | | | | | | | | | | | | | | | | |
| STOP | | | | | | | | | | | | | | | | | | | |
| START | ℞ No. | | 1 | 2 | 3 | 4 | 5 | 6 | 7 | 8 | 9 | 10 | 11 | 12 | 13 | 14 | 15 | 16 | |
| RENEW | | | 17 | 18 | 19 | 20 | 21 | 22 | 23 | 24 | 25 | 26 | 27 | 28 | 29 | 30 | 31 | | |
| STOP | | | | | | | | | | | | | | | | | | | |
| START | ℞ No. | | 1 | 2 | 3 | 4 | 5 | 6 | 7 | 8 | 9 | 10 | 11 | 12 | 13 | 14 | 15 | 16 | |
| RENEW | | | 17 | 18 | 19 | 20 | 21 | 22 | 23 | 24 | 25 | 26 | 27 | 28 | 29 | 30 | 31 | | |
| STOP | | | | | | | | | | | | | | | | | | | |
| START | ℞ No. | | 1 | 2 | 3 | 4 | 5 | 6 | 7 | 8 | 9 | 10 | 11 | 12 | 13 | 14 | 15 | 16 | |
| RENEW | | | 17 | 18 | 19 | 20 | 21 | 22 | 23 | 24 | 25 | 26 | 27 | 28 | 29 | 30 | 31 | | |
| STOP | | | | | | | | | | | | | | | | | | | |
| START | ℞ No. | | 1 | 2 | 3 | 4 | 5 | 6 | 7 | 8 | 9 | 10 | 11 | 12 | 13 | 14 | 15 | 16 | |
| RENEW | | | 17 | 18 | 19 | 20 | 21 | 22 | 23 | 24 | 25 | 26 | 27 | 28 | 29 | 30 | 31 | | |
| STOP | | | | | | | | | | | | | | | | | | | |
| START | ℞ No. | | 1 | 2 | 3 | 4 | 5 | 6 | 7 | 8 | 9 | 10 | 11 | 12 | 13 | 14 | 15 | 16 | |
| RENEW | | | 17 | 18 | 19 | 20 | 21 | 22 | 23 | 24 | 25 | 26 | 27 | 28 | 29 | 30 | 31 | | |
| STOP | | | | | | | | | | | | | | | | | | | |
| START | ℞ No. | | 1 | 2 | 3 | 4 | 5 | 6 | 7 | 8 | 9 | 10 | 11 | 12 | 13 | 14 | 15 | 16 | |
| RENEW | | | 17 | 18 | 19 | 20 | 21 | 22 | 23 | 24 | 25 | 26 | 27 | 28 | 29 | 30 | 31 | | |
| STOP | | | | | | | | | | | | | | | | | | | |
| START | ℞ No. | | 1 | 2 | 3 | 4 | 5 | 6 | 7 | 8 | 9 | 10 | 11 | 12 | 13 | 14 | 15 | 16 | |
| RENEW | | | 17 | 18 | 19 | 20 | 21 | 22 | 23 | 24 | 25 | 26 | 27 | 28 | 29 | 30 | 31 | | |
| STOP | | | | | | | | | | | | | | | | | | | |
| START | ℞ No. | | 1 | 2 | 3 | 4 | 5 | 6 | 7 | 8 | 9 | 10 | 11 | 12 | 13 | 14 | 15 | 16 | |
| RENEW | | | 17 | 18 | 19 | 20 | 21 | 22 | 23 | 24 | 25 | 26 | 27 | 28 | 29 | 30 | 31 | | |
| STOP | | | | | | | | | | | | | | | | | | | |

PATIENT NO. _____     FLOOR _____

ALLERGY _____     ROOM _____

PATIENT _____

DIAGNOSIS _____

DOCTOR _____

29

# Dispensing

A pharmacist or a trained technician performs the actual dispensing of medication.

A method of checking the medication after dispensing must be used. The check is preferably made by someone other than the person dispensing. The type of drug distribution system in use may determine the exact procedure used for the final check. If a nonpharmacist (state regulations permitting) dispenses, a pharmacist must make the final check regardless of the distribution system. If a unit dose system is used, dispensing is often performed from an order sheet such as that pictured in Fig. 3-7. PRN medications are included on the reverse side.

## Labeling

The prescription label may have specific and unique requirements depending upon the facility's policies, drug distribution system, and whether a computer system is used. The prescription label must coincide with the drug order instructions. The label must also provide the facility staff with additional information that will help ensure that the right drug is administered to the right patient at the right time. Good label preparation procedures should include arrangement of the basic information on the prescription label in a specific format.

In this way, the label will always have the same format no matter how many different pharmacy employees are responsible for label preparation. This procedure helps the facility staff to read the label more efficiently.

All names of medications should be spelled out except where the pharmaceutical services committee has established a list of approved abbreviations. The directions should be as specific as possible and always include the strength of the medication if the drug has one. If the dose to be administered is different from the drug strength, the directions should always indicate the volume (number of milliliters) or quantity (e.g., ½ tablet) that is equivalent to the dose to be administered.

When identifying a drug on the label by its generic name, the pharmacist should indicate the manufacturer's name on the label. Many states require this.

Additional auxiliary label information may be included on the main prescription label or may be added to the container at the time of dispensing. Auxiliary label information usually includes additional or specific storage requirements, specific administration procedures to follow, and reorder information when appropriate. The use of an auxiliary label is a method of direct communication with the facility staff, using the specific knowledge of the pharmacist about the proper storage, administration, and overall handling of medications in the drug distribution system. Figure 3-8 shows an example of prescription labeling procedures and a prescription label using the traditional system.

Some states allow the directions for administration to be written in the Medication Administration Record (MAR), rather than on the label. In this case, the pharmacy prepares the MAR with the directions. If directions change during the course of therapy, a new MAR is prepared.

## Formulary

A formulary system is the process by which the medical staff, through the pharmaceutical services committee evaluates and selects from the numerous drug products available those it considers to be most useful to patient care in its institution. The formulary itself is the vehicle by which the medical and nursing staffs make use of the system. The formulary system is one part of a program of objective evaluation, selection, and use of medicinal agents in the institution to promote rational drug therapy and a cost-effective operation.

The formulary system may limit the brands, dosage forms, and strengths of a particular drug entity for use in the institution. It may limit the drug entities to be used within various classes of drugs, such as use of one particular thiazide diuretic. When an institutional formulary is in use, the medical staff agrees to limit the use of drugs to those approved for inclusion in the formulary. Use of the formulary system includes procedures for additions and other changes in the formulary.

**Figure 3-8**

# Example of Medication Labeling Procedures Used for an Individual Prescription System

All legend patient medication regardless of the source will be properly labeled. The nurse receiving the drugs assumes the responsibility for assuring that all items coming from the pharmacy are properly labeled. *Any item labeled improperly should be rejected and returned to the originating pharmacy.*

Drug containers having soiled, damaged, incomplete, illegible, or makeshift labels will be returned to the issuing pharmacists or pharmacy for relabeling or disposal. Drugs in containers having no labels will be destroyed in accordance with state and federal laws.

The drug label should not be altered, modified, or marked in any way by a nurse resulting in any change of the original. If necessary, a "signal" type label should be placed on the prescription indicating that there has been a change in the order affecting the administration of the drug and that the nurse should turn to the patient's health record for more correct information.

Labels must be affixed to, not inserted in, vials, since insertion in the vial facilitates removal and greatly increases the risk of error.

## A PRESCRIPTION LABEL

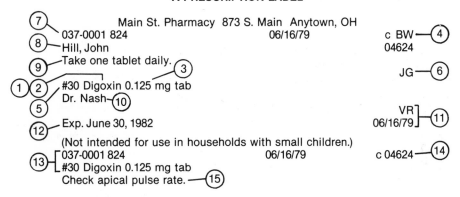

1. Trade name, where appropriate.
2. Name of medication.
3. Strength of medication when appropriate.
4. Manufacturer, when appropriate.
5. Quantity.
6. Initial of pharmacist.
7. Prescription number.
8. Patient's name, last name first.
9. Directions.
10. Physician's name.
11. Date prescription dispensed and initial of typist.
12. Expiration date of medication.
13. Reorder strip.
14. Patient's facility admission number.
15. Auxiliary instruction strip.

Some states have established formularies as part of the state's drug product selection law. In other states, such legislation requires pharmacists to establish their own formularies. Formularies established for long-term care facilities must be consistent with these laws.

Long-term care facilities may experience difficulty in establishing a formulary system because it must be adopted and used by the medical staff. Physicians serving long-term care facilities are usually community-based and may not abide by a formulary. In spite of these difficulties, some pharmacists have successfully implemented formulary systems in the long-term care facilities they serve. Success depends on the relationship between the pharmacist and the facility staff. A good formulary system can contribute to better patient care and allow economical purchasing by the pharmacist because of the limitation on products required to be stocked. A good formulary should also provide a mechanism to obtain non-formulary drugs when specific indications require it.

# DELIVERY OF DRUGS

*Pharmacist's Responsibilities*

- Determines necessity of immediately handling the preparation and delivery of the medication to the patient (emergency or stat)
- Establishes and monitors a system to ensure proper storage conditions for perishable items during delivery
- Develops and maintains a record keeping system to account for drugs dispensed from the pharmacy and received by the facility

## Procedures

As drug orders are prepared, they should be placed in a specific holding area prior to delivery to the facility or nursing unit.

The drug distribution system used may have specific types of equipment for transportation of completed orders. No matter what the system or equipment, all orders going to the facility should be clearly marked and identified to indicate the facility and the nursing station to which they are to be delivered. Before deliveries leave the pharmacy, a final check should be made to ensure that the order is complete, that all back-orders are accounted for or noted. If an order requires special handling, a separate slip or form should be attached to the order highlighting the special instructions. A security system should be developed to assure that orders are delivered intact.

Stat or emergency orders should have priority. Some states have specific time parameters for stat or emergency deliveries. Appropriate procedures should be developed to ensure that the patient's needs are met and all state and federal regulations are adhered to.

If the pharmacy is located some distance from the facility, a pharmacy near the facility may be used on a contract basis to provide stat or emergency services. A delivery schedule and route schedule should be developed. The facility staff should know approximately when the pharmacy delivery and pick-ups will be made on a daily basis. A delivery schedule is also helpful in scheduling pharmacy personnel.

Drug orders should never be left at a facility without having the authorized facility personnel sign for or acknowledge the receipt of an order. Figure 3-9 is an example of a form used to record drugs delivered and acknowledge their receipt. Orders should not be left unattended at a nursing station. Appropriate procedures for delivery of drugs to nursing units should be developed whether the pharmacy is on- or off-premises.

Figure 3-9

# Pharmacy

PHARMACY USE ONLY

No. Orders_____ Pharmacy Chart_____

Date_____ Pharmacy Filling_____

Facility_____ No._____ Station_____ Ordered By_____

The Facility Acknowledges Receipt of All Items Listed. ☐ As Form is Amended.

Signature:_____ Date_____ Date_____

ALL RX's - COMPLETE ALL COLUMNS.

| Pharm. Use | Patient's Name | Pat. No. | Ph. Order | Item Rec'd | Comments | Medication Name & Strength | Directions | Physician |
|---|---|---|---|---|---|---|---|---|
| | | | | | | | | |
| | | | | | | | | |
| | | | | | | | | |
| | | | | | | | | |
| | | | | | | | | |
| | | | | | | | | |
| | | | | | | | | |
| | | | | | | | | |
| | | | | | | | | |
| | | | | | | | | |
| | | | | | | | | |
| | | | | | | | | |

PHARMACY MEDICATION ORDER

# STORAGE

*Pharmacist's Responsibilities*

- Establishes and monitors a system to ensure proper storage conditions from receipt in the pharmacy to administration to the patient or destruction of the medication
- Develops a system to make emergency medications available, including an emergency kit
- Develops a system to replace quickly medication from the emergency kit when it is used or expired

## Procedures

Drugs are stored in the pharmacy prior to dispensing and at the nursing units prior to administration. Whether the pharmacy is on- or off-premises, it must adhere to state and federal laws and regulations concerning storage and physical facilities. Regulations also dictate storage requirements at the nursing units.

In both the pharmacy and at the nursing unit, drugs for external use should be stored separately from drugs for internal use. Test reagents, germicides, disinfectants, and other household substances should be stored separately from drugs. The USP requirements concerning storage temperatures apply in the nursing unit as well as the pharmacy. Room temperature is defined as not less than 15 °C or more than 30 °C (59–86 °F). Drugs requiring storage in a "cool place" are stored at a temperature between 2 °C (36 °F) and 15 °C (59 °F).

If drugs are stored in the same refrigerator with food, the drugs must be kept in a closed, properly labeled container. If the refrigerator is not located in a locked medication room, the box containing the medications must be locked.

At the nursing unit, all medications are stored in a locked cabinet, cart, or room inaccessible to patients and visitors. Drugs should be stored in an orderly manner in cabinets, drawers, or on shelves of sufficient size to prevent crowding. State laws and regulations may specify the dimensions required. Dose preparation and dispensing areas should be well lighted. Only personnel designated in writing by the pharmaceutical services policies should have access to drugs. In the case of an on-premises pharmacy, only the pharmacist should have a key to the pharmacy. At the nursing unit, only the charge nurse or designee should have the key to the medication storage unit.

Drugs for each patient are stored in the containers in which they were dispensed. Drugs should not be transferred to containers other than those in which they were dispensed by anyone other than a pharmacist. Each patient's drugs should be stored in an individually labeled compartment. All drugs on hand for patients who expire, and those drugs not sent home with patients at the time of discharge, must be immediately withdrawn from stock and either locked away or destroyed in conformance with the drug destruction procedure. State regulations may specify procedures to be used in drug destruction.

The locked drug storage area may be a cabinet, room, or cart. The drug cart is an integral part of some drug distribution systems, particularly the unit dose system and the blister card modification of the traditional system. The carts usually consist of removable components in which the drugs are placed. The drawers or trays are "filled" in the pharmacy, delivered to the nursing unit, and interchanged with the "used" drawers or trays. The cart itself may be locked or kept in a locked room. The carts are designed to meet all requirements for security and separation of drugs. Carts are owned either by the pharmacy or the facility. When the facility owns the cart, it is then committed to use the drug distribution system compatible with the equipment it owns regardless of the pharmaceutical service provider.

## Emergency Kits

The purpose of maintaining emergency kits at each nursing station is to provide immediate access to drugs that might be needed in a life-threatening situation. Emergency drugs are primarily for the treatment of cardiac arrest, circulatory collapse, allergic reaction, convulsions, and bronchial spasms. They are generally parenteral medications. All drugs should be issued as near ready as possible for administration. The emergency drug kit should not be a source for normal "PRN" drug orders. The pharmaceutical services committee determines the drugs to be stocked in the emergency kits. An example of the drugs contained in an emergency kit is shown in Fig. 3-10.

## Figure 3-10 — Contents of Emergency Kit

| DRUG | SIZE | QUANTITY | DRAWER | THERAPEUTIC CLASSIFICATION |
|------|------|----------|--------|----------------------------|
| ADRENALIN 1:1000 | 1cc | 3 | 6 | VASOPRESSOR, BRONCHODILATOR |
| ALIDASE | AMP | 3 | 7 | HYALURONIDASE |
| * AMINOPHYLLINE IM 250 mg/10 cc | 10cc | 2 | 6 | CARDIAC STIMULANT, BRONCHODILATOR |
| * AMINOPHYLLINE IV 500 mg/2 cc | 2cc | 2 | 6 | CARDIAC STIMULANT, BRONCHODILATOR |
| * ARAMINE 1% | 1cc | 3 | 10 | VASOPRESSOR |
| ATROPINE SULFATE 0.4 mg/cc | 1cc | 3 | 12 | ANTISPASMODIC |
| * AQUA-MEPHYTON 10 mg/cc | 1cc | 3 | 9 | VITAMIN K |
| BENADRYL 50 mg/cc | 1cc | 3 | 9 | ANTIHISTAMINE |
| CAFFEINE/SOD. BENZOATE 500 mg/2 cc | 2cc | 3 | 12 | ANALEPTIC (CNS STIMULANT) |
| * CALCIUM GLUCONATE 10% | 10cc | 1 | 10 | CALCIUM REPLACEMENT |
| COMPAZINE 5 mg/cc | 2cc | 3 | 1 | ANTIEMETIC |
| * CEDILANID-D 0.4 mg/2 cc | 2cc | 3 | 8 | CARDIAC STIMULANT |
| CORAMINE 25% | 1.5cc | 3 | 12 | ANALEPTIC (CNS STIMULANT) |
| * DECADRON 4 mg/cc | 1cc | 1 | 13 | ANTIINFLAMMATORY |
| * DEXTROSE 50% | 50cc | 1 | 13 | CARBOHYDRATE REPLACEMENT |
| * DIGITOXIN 0.2 mg/cc | 1cc | 3 | 8 | CARDIAC STIMULANT |
| DIGOXIN (LANOXIN) 0.25 mg/cc | 2cc | 3 | 8 | CARDIAC STIMULANT |
| DILANTIN (100 mg/amp) | AMP | 1 | 5 | ANTICONVULSANT |
| * GLUCAGON 1.0 mg/amp | AMP | 1 | 7 | HYPOGLYCEMIC SHOCK (INSULIN SHOCK) |
| * HEPARIN 40,000 U/cc | 2cc | 1 | 8 | ANTICOAGULANT |
| * ISUPREL 1:5000/cc | 1cc | 3 | 6 | BRONCHODILATOR |
| KENALOG IM 40 mg/cc | 1cc | 1 | 7 | ANTIINFLAMMATORY |
| LASIX 10 mg/cc | 2cc | 4 | 9 | DIURETIC |
| * LEVOPHED 2 mg/cc | 4cc | 1 | 10 | VASOPRESSOR |
| MAGNESIUM SULFATE 50% | 2cc | 3 | 5 | ANTICONVULSANT |
| * PHENERGAN 50 mg/cc | 1cc | 3 | 11 | ANTIEMETIC, TRANQUILIZER |
| PHENOBARBITAL 2 gr/amp | AMP | 3 | 5 | ANTICONVULSANT, SEDATIVE |
| * POTASSIUM CHLORIDE 40 meq/amp | AMP | 1 | 13 | POTASSIUM REPLACEMENT |
| QUINIDINE SULFATE 80 mg/cc | 1cc | 3 | 10 | ANTIARRHYTHMIC (HEART) |
| SERPASIL 2.5 mg/cc | 2cc | 2 | 12 | ANTIHYPERTENSIVE |
| SODIUM BICARBONATE 7.5% 44.6 meq/50 cc | 50cc | 1 | 13 | SYSTEMIC ACIDOSIS (ALKALINIZER) |
| * SYNKAYVITE 75 mg/2 cc | 2cc | 2 | 9 | VITAMIN K |
| THORAZINE 25 mg/cc | 2cc | 3 | 11 | TRANQUILIZER, ANTIEMETIC |
| * TIGAN 200 mg/2 cc | 2cc | 3 | 1 | ANTIEMETIC |
| * VISTARIL 50 mg/cc | 2cc | 3 | 11 | TRANQUILIZER |
| WATER FOR INJECTION | 30cc | 1 | 13 | DILUENT |
| XYLOCAINE 2% | 2cc | 2 | 7 | ANESTHETIC (LOCAL) |

* DATED ITEM

(This is one example of the contents of the Emergency Kit in a long-term care facility. These kits sometimes contain injectable antibiotics in addition to the drug categories listed.)

The emergency kit is sealed with an expiration date of not more than 1 year—often less—due to the instability of certain drugs contained in them. Although some state regulations require that the kit be kept in a locked cabinet, in general the kit should not be locked to allow for easy access. Since the kit is sealed, it is obvious when it has been opened. As soon as the kit is opened for any reason, it should be returned to the pharmacist to be restocked and reissued. Some pharmacists keep an extra stocked kit in the pharmacy to hasten the exchange process. There is not a specific requirement for the type of container that may be used as an emergency kit. Pharmacists have used various styles of plastic boxes and fishing tackle boxes.

Pharmacists sometimes encounter problems in maintaining sealed kits in the facility because nursing personnel neglect to inform the pharmacist each time a kit is used. To alleviate this problem, kits have been designed that may be opened without a key but require a key for closing and resealing. The presence of an opened kit, which absolutely cannot be reclosed without a key, serves as a reminder to facility staff to call the pharmacist each time the kit is used. The pharmacist should inspect kits regularly to be sure no doses have expired and that they are completely stocked. The forms shown in Fig. 3-11 and 3-12 assist the pharmacist in checking the kits for expired drugs.

Drugs are arranged in the kit to permit visibility and ease of selection. A list of the contents should be posted near the telephone since emergency telephone orders may be given by the physician. Another list should be placed inside the sealed kit. A requisition form (Fig. 3-13) may be placed inside to record administered drugs. The drugs administered should also be recorded in the patient's record. It is important for the pharmacist to know the identity and location of the patient who received the drugs both for the purposes of drug therapy monitoring and for appropriate billing.

**Figure 3-11**

**THE EMERGENCY DRUG KIT**
NOTICE:
FOR EMERGENCY USE ONLY

THIS SEAL MAY BE BROKEN
ONLY ON THE ORDER OF
A PHYSICIAN

STOCKED AND SEALED BY

_____
Signature of Consulting Pharmacist

_____
Expiration Date

After each use or immediately prior
to expiration date, return this kit to

**PHARMACY**
to be restocked

Figure 3-12
## EMERGENCY KIT EXPIRATION DATES

DRAWER ONE
TIGAN _1-97_
COMPAZINE _2-93_
DRAMAMINE ___

DRAWER TWO
PENICILLIN G _11-86_
TERRAMYCIN _9-79_
AMPICILLIN _8-83_
GARAMYCIN _1-86_

DRAWER THREE
LINCOCIN _2-91_
KEFLIN _9-87_
LORIDINE _11-87_
KANTREX _9-91_

DRAWER FOUR
TERRAMYCIN IV _6-79_
TETRACYCLINE IM _6-86_
TETRACYCLINE IV ___
TALWIN ___

DRAWER FIVE
DILANTIN ___
MAG. SULFATE ___
LUMINAL ___

DRAWER SIX
ISUPREL ___
AMINOPHYLLINE IM ___
AMINOPHYLLINE IV ___
ADRENALIN ___

DRAWER SEVEN
GLUCAGON ___
ALIDASE ___
KENALOG ___
XYLOCAINE ___

DRAWER EIGHT
LANOXIN ___
HEPARIN ___
CEDILANID-D ___
CRYSTODIGIN ___

DRAWER NINE
AQUAMEPHYTON ___
LASIX ___
LORFAN ___
BENADRYL ___
SYNKAYVITE ___

DRAWER TEN
QUINIDINE SULF ___
ARAMINE ___
CALCIUM GLUCONATE ___
LEVOPHED ___

DRAWER ELEVEN
VALIUM ___
THORAZINE ___
VISTARIL ___
PHENERGAN ___

DRAWER TWELVE
CORAMINE ___
SERPASIL ___
CAFFEINE & SOD. BENZOATE ___
ATROPINE ___

DRAWER THIRTEEN
SOD. BICARBONATE ___
DECADRON ___
BACTERIOSTATIC WATER ___
POTASSIUM CHLORIDE ___
DEXTROSE ___

ADDITIONAL COMMENTS:

**Figure 3-13**

A.                              ITEM(S) USED FROM EMERGENCY KIT

DATE: _____

FACILITY: _____

STATION: _____

PATIENT: _____

ITEM(S) USED: _____ _____

_____

_____

_____

_____

B.                              EMERGENCY KIT RECORD

KIT NO. _____

| DATE STOCKED | EXP. DATE | DATE SENT | FACILITY & STATION | DATE USED | ITEM | DATE RETURNED |
|---|---|---|---|---|---|---|
|  |  |  |  |  |  |  |
|  |  |  |  |  |  |  |
|  |  |  |  |  |  |  |
|  |  |  |  |  |  |  |

## Stat and PRN Drug Supplies

A few states allow the use of "stat boxes" in long-term care facilities. The stat medication cabinet is used for new orders, changed medication orders, and replacement for missing or damaged medication for regularly scheduled drugs.

This supply consists of the most frequently ordered medications. The number of different drugs and strengths of a single drug to be placed in the stat medication cabinet is determined by the pharmaceutical services committee. The committee determines the amount of stock needed by studying how frequently such medications are used. State regulations that allow the use of these supplies generally place an upper limit on the number of doses of any specific drug, such as a maximum of six doses, usually supplied in unit dose packaging. Use of a stat box requires special record keeping so that all drugs used are accounted for and an accurate record of the patient's drug regimen is maintained. The stat box may be the only expedient source of the first dose of drugs, such as antiinfectives, antipyretics, antinauseants, analgesics, and antidiarrheals for the waiting patient when the pharmacist is not immediately available.

# ACCOUNTABILITY

*Pharmacist's Responsibilities*

- Develops and maintains an inventory system for all drugs and pharmaceutical supplies for active and inactive storage areas
- Assists in design and implementation of record systems for use in the pharmacy (e.g., patient records, inventory control, and drug utilization)
- Develops and implements an appropriate security system to prevent theft and/or drug diversion
- Maintains a record of controlled substances received, stored, and dispensed by the pharmacy and administered in the facility
- Develops and maintains a system for regular removal from storage areas of all pharmaceutical items that are outdated or whose manufacture has been discontinued

## Procedures

The use and disposition of all drugs supplied to the long-term care facility should be documented in the patients' health records and other appropriate facility records. Certain drugs such as controlled substances require special control and accountability procedures.

## Controlled Substances

The Drug Enforcement Administration regulates labeling, handling, and accountability of narcotics, sedatives, stimulants, and other drugs with abuse potential in compliance with the Controlled Substances Act of 1970. The controlled narcotics, sedatives, and hypnotics are listed in five schedules indicating potential for abuse.

Long-term care facilities are not eligible for registration with the Drug Enforcement Administration and may not possess controlled substances. Any controlled drugs present in the facility should have been dispensed pursuant to a prescription for a particular patient. Federal regulations concerning controlled substances in LTCFs are contained in the Medicare and Medicaid standards.

Drugs listed in Schedules II, III, and IV of the Drug Abuse Prevention and Control Act must not be accessible to other than licensed nursing, pharmacy, and medical personnel designated by the facility. The director of nursing service is usually designated by the facility to be responsible for the control of such drugs. Controlled substances ordered by the physician should be sent in easily accountable quantities. Controlled parenteral substances should be sent in the smallest available dosage unit, preferably unit dose. Multidose vials should not be sent except in emergency situations and where unit dose is not available. No medication which requires a written prescription, such as those in Schedule II, should be delivered until the prescription is in the facility or in the hands of the pharmacist. All Schedule II controlled substances are stored under double lock, separate from all other medications.

Separate records must be maintained on all Schedule II drugs. Such records must be accurate and include: the name of the patient, name of the prescriber, prescription number, drug name, form of the medication, strength and dose administered, date and time of administration, and signature of the person administering the drug. Such records regularly are reconciled to a physical count of the remaining doses and are retained at least 2 years. Drug records are maintained for drugs listed in Schedules III and IV to trace the receipt and disposition of such drugs.

## Investigational Drugs

Some long-term care facilities have policies that allow the use of investigational drugs. Such drugs require special procedures to assure that their use complies with state and federal laws and accepted professional principles.

In general, investigational drugs may be administered to patients in the facility providing the following conditions are met:

- The patient and the patient's responsible party have signed all of the various releases required by state and federal law.
- The patient care policy committee has reviewed and approved the use of a specific drug or treatment for a specific patient.
- All requirements of the various agencies that control such drugs are met.
- Information on the drug is supplied to the pharmacist responsible for monitoring the patient's drug regimen.

Further information on use of investigational drugs in the long-term care facility may be obtained from the Food and Drug Administration, Division of Scientific Investigations, Institutional Review Board Branch (HFD-180), 5600 Fishers Lane, Rockville, Maryland 20857.

## Drug Disposal

Disposal of drugs is any process by which a substance leaves or is removed from the drug area, the facility, or any other storage area maintained by the facility, except for authorized administration to a patient. Discontinued, excess, or expired drugs should be removed by the pharmacist and disposed appropriately. Requirements for drug disposal vary among the states. Some state regulations allow the pharmacist to destroy drugs in the presence of authorized witnesses, such as licensed nurses or the facility surveyor. The pharmacist should keep a drug disposition record which includes the name of the patient, the name and strength of drugs destroyed, date of destruction, and the signatures of the pharmacist and witnesses.

Occasionally, a drug will be discontinued with a good possibility of its reorder, e.g., drugs used in chronic urinary tract infections. In such cases, the pharmacist may hold the discontinued drug in reserve for a limited time and reissue it as an economic courtesy to the patient. One procedure is to mark the containers of discontinued drugs to indicate the date of discontinuation. Discontinued drugs are then disposed of within 90 days of the date of discontinuation, unless the drug is reordered within that time.

All drugs provided by a pharmacist on prescription of a physician should be destroyed when the patient is discharged or deceased. Drugs belonging to deceased persons should never be sent with personal belongings to the mortuary. If the physician wishes a drug to be sent home or transferred with a discharged patient, he or she must write such an order. The prescription must be labeled as an outpatient prescription. Controlled drugs may be sent with the patient on discharge if ordered by the discharging physician. An entry must be made in the facility's controlled substances inventory record to indicate disposition of the drugs.

Discontinued controlled substances pose a particular problem in LTCFs due to conflicting opinions concerning their disposal. If a patient no longer requires the controlled drug(s), the facility should have written procedures to deal with their disposition in accordance with applicable regulations. If these drugs may be destroyed at the facility, the pharmacist may destroy them in the presence of the nurse and document the fact on the patient's medical record. It is advisable to check with the appropriate state agency(ies) for direction.

Drug discards due to discontinued and expired drugs represent a significant cost in providing pharmaceutical service. Many pharmacists using unit dose distribution systems have requested state agencies to allow return of unused medication to inventory for reuse. They argue that the medication has not been removed from its original package and so retains its integrity for reuse. However, most states will not allow reuse of medications, regardless of the packaging system. When a unit dose system is used, however, the quantity of medication dispensed at one time is small. Therefore, relatively little medication is wasted if the drug is discontinued. Pharmacists using traditional distribution systems have found that imposing stop orders or limited quantity dispensing on drugs which are usually used for short periods decreases waste.

## References for Further Reading

Berman, R. S., "Mobile Unit Dose System Simplifies Distribution of Drugs and Reduces Errors," *Modern Nursing Home, 24*, 24(March 1970).

Crawley, H. K. and F. M. Eckel, "Comparison of a Traditional and Unit Dose Drug Distribution System in a Nursing Home," *Drug Intell. Clin. Pharm., 5*, 166(1971).

*Developing, Maintaining and Using Patient Medication Profiles*, Academy of Pharmacy Practice, American Pharmaceutical Association, Washington, D.C., 1975.

Farner, J. and C. Hicks, "The Impact of Drug Distribution Systems on Nurses' Time Involvement in Medication Related Activities in Long-Term Care Facilities," *Drug Intell. Clin. Pharm., 10*, 458(1976).

"Guidelines for Repackaging Oral Solids and Liquids in Single Unit and Unit Dose Packages," *Am. J. Hosp. Pharm., 34*, 1355(1977).

"Guidelines for Single Unit and Unit Dose Packages of Drugs," *Am. J. Hosp. Pharm., 34*, 613(1977).

Mathieson, D. R. and J. L. Rawlings, "Evaluation of a Unit Dose System in Nursing Homes as Implemented by a Community Pharmacy," *Am. J. Hosp. Pharm., 28*, 254(1971).

Minor, M., "Justifying the Cost of a Unit Dose System Without Reliance on Savings for Nursing," *Hosp. Pharm., 10*, 94(March 1975).

Patry, R. A. and R. Kroeger, "Drug Waste and Prescribing in Two Nursing Homes," *Contemp. Pharm. Pract., 1*, 28(1978).

Rawlings, J. L. and P. A. Frisk, "Pharmaceutical Services in SNFs in Compliance with Federal Regulations," *Am. J. Hosp. Pharm., 32*, 905(1975).

Reamer, J. T. *et al.*, "Moisture Permeation of Typical Unit Dose Repackaging Materials," *Am. J. Hosp. Pharm., 34*, 42(1977).

Relyea, K. D., "Nursing Home Pharmacy: Unit Dose Solves Problems Unique to Nursing Homes," *Modern Nursing Home, 26*, 12(1971).

*Sourcebook on Unit Dose Drug Distribution Systems*, American Society of Hospital Pharmacists, Washington, D.C., 1978.

"Statement on Unit Dose Drug Distribution Systems," *Am. J. Hosp. Pharm., 32*, 835(1975).

*Unit Dose Implementation Manual*, Abbott Laboratories, North Chicago, Ill., 1975.

Watt, J., "Chronic Care Facility and the Community Pharmacist," *Can. Pharm. J., 109*, 167(1976).

Weimann, W. *et al.*, "Unit Dose—A Challenge to the Claim of Cost Effectiveness in SNFs," *Calif. Pharm., 24*, 42(April 1976).

# Chapter 4:
# NONDISPENSING SERVICES

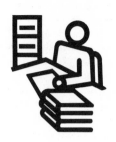

Nondispensing services cover functions performed by pharmacists that are not immediately associated with dispensing medications to patients (see Fig. 2-1). They begin with drug administration to the patient and are followed by drug regimen review, the pharmacist's committee participation, and provision of inservice education and patient counselling. These services may be viewed as the pharmacist's responsibility to assure appropriate results through drug therapy monitoring, establishment of policies and procedures, and education.

## ADMINISTRATION OF DRUGS

*Pharmacist's Responsibilities*

Although the pharmacist may not usually administer medications, he or she should be concerned with administration procedures. Correct administration is crucial to the success of drug therapy and is an integral part of the medication system. The pharmacist should participate in the development of policies and procedures for drug administration. The procedures should specify correct administration procedures and a system for detecting, recording, and monitoring drug administration errors.

### Procedures

The eight "rights" referred to at the beginning of Chapter 2 in connection with the medication system also apply to the activities of drug administration. The person administering medications incorporates the eight rights into the procedures as follows:

*Right Patient*
- Checks the band on the patient's wrist.
- Asks the patient his or her name.

*Right Drug*
- Reads the drug order on the drug administration form (drug sheets or drug administration record).

*Right Dose*
- Reads the dosage as ordered on the drug administration form.
- Reads the dosage indicated on the prescription label.

*Right Dosage Form and Right Route of Administration*
- Reads the route ordered on the drug administration form.
- Checks the dosage form of the drug.

*Right Time*
- Reads the administration time as indicated on the drug administration form.
- Administers at the indicated time.

*Right Record*
- Records date, time, initials of person administering, dose, and drug administered after administration.

*Right Response*
- Observes patient's immediate response to drug.

In most states, only licensed personnel are assigned responsibility for preparing, administering, and recording of drugs or have access to drug storage areas at each nursing station. Drugs should always be prepared and administered by the same person. Drugs supplied for one patient must not be administered to another patient. Patients must not be allowed to self-administer *any* drug unless specifically ordered to do so by their attending physician, except as prohibited by state regulations. Drug administration errors and untoward drug reactions should be reported immediately to the attending physician, charted in detail on the nurse's notes, and described on an incident report. Personnel administering drugs should refer to a good reference or request information from the pharmacist when unfamiliar with the pharmacology of the drug, its potential toxic effects, and contraindications. Current references should be available at each nursing unit. The pharmacist is also responsible for providing additional drug information as needed. The facility should provide an adequate supply of disposable containers for the administration of drugs. No disposable container used in the administration of drugs should be re-used.

In addition to the preceding procedures, all inventoried controlled drugs must be counted by licensed personnel routinely. A record of this count is entered on the medication nurse's log. Each completed medication nurse's log sheet is forwarded to the Director of Nursing Service and retained for a time defined by the facility's policies.

## Medication System Error List

The facility should maintain a medication system error list in order to:
- Establish a procedure of monitoring and keeping a record of errors which may occur through the source of supply or in the administration of drugs.
- Assist the pharmacy providers to perfect their service by keeping an organized record of errors originating with them.
- Bring problem areas to the attention of the pharmacist for guidance and assistance.

The director of nursing service should instruct licensed nursing personnel to enter any problems or errors they observe in the medication system, take appropriate action to have errors corrected, and enter the information in the log. Serious errors should be brought to the attention of the director, or his or her relief, immediately. The director, or the relief person, should check the log on a regular basis to ensure that appropriate action is being taken to correct any errors. An Incident Report on each error should be filled out and sent to the Administrator. An example of a form for this medication error list is given in Fig. 4-1. The pharmacist should monitor the incidence of drug administration errors and use this information in diagnosing and correcting any problems the facility may have regarding drug administration procedures.

*The following is an example of one facility's drug administration procedures.*

In a distribution system in which a drug cart is used, the refrigerated items are placed on the cart before the pass begins. All drugs are given and charted immediately. If a patient is not in his or her room, or otherwise not available, a clip is attached to the drug sheet to indicate that the patient has not received the drugs. When the pass is completed, the nurse may return and give the patient the drugs.

During the routine drug administration pass, the cart is brought to the patient's bedside for the administration and charting procedure. If this is impossible, the cart is brought to the doorway of the patient's room with the drawers facing inward. When PRN doses or odd hour doses are administered, other than during routine pass, it is not necessary to take the cart to the patient's room or bedside. The PRN or odd hour dose is prepared at the site of the cart storage area and the dose(s) is taken to the patient, leaving the cart secured in the cart storage area.

All drugs are listed on a drug sheet. The drug sheets are treated as a "kardex." Any change in physician's instructions is immediately recorded on this sheet. Drug cards are not used in this system. The record keeping procedure consists of direct charting. Charting is done immediately after giving the patient the drug, before going on to the next patient. In the space provided on the drug sheet, the nurse indicates the time the dose was actually administered and the site of any injections administered. All PRNs and refusals are charted in

Figure 4-1

## MEDICATION SYSTEM ERROR LIST

| DATE | PATIENT NAME | WHAT HAPPENED? | WHO NOTICED IT? | WHAT ACTION WAS TAKEN TO CORRECT IT? |
|------|--------------|----------------|-----------------|--------------------------------------|
|      |              |                |                 |                                      |
|      |              |                |                 |                                      |
|      |              |                |                 |                                      |
|      |              |                |                 |                                      |
|      |              |                |                 |                                      |
|      |              |                |                 |                                      |
|      |              |                |                 |                                      |
|      |              |                |                 |                                      |
|      |              |                |                 |                                      |
|      |              |                |                 |                                      |
|      |              |                |                 |                                      |
|      |              |                |                 |                                      |

the appropriate space on the back of the sheet. If further charting is required in the nurses' notes, a clip is placed on the drug sheet and the entries made in the nurses' notes immediately after the pass is completed, using the clips as reminders. The controlled substances proof of use sheets accompany the cart and signing-off a dose is done at the time the drug is administered, as well as charting on the drug sheet.

The nurse administering the drugs is responsible for charting. Charting is completed as soon as possible following drug administration. The nurse responsible for drugs must not report off-duty without first completing charting. Subsequent administration intervals depend on these recordings. Each dose should be initialed on the daily drug report after administration. The nurse verifies the initial with her or his full signature and title in the space provided on the administration record.

Drugs given on an as needed basis (PRN) are recorded on the back of the sheet in addition to the normal charting procedure, including:

1. The patient's subjective symptoms or complaints.
2. The dose, time, route of administration, and, if appropriate, the injection site.
3. The results.
4. The nurse's signature.

Example:

1/1/70, 1:50 p.m., Demerol 50 mg, p.o., given for nagging pain in left shoulder, with relief.                       B. Y. Jingo, RN

If a dose of regular interval drug is withheld or regurgitated, the nurse's initial for the dose in question is circled. A full explanatory note is written in the record area where PRN recordings are made.

Figure 4-2 illustrates the record forms that are used.

# REVIEW OF DRUG REGIMEN

*Pharmacist's Responsibilities*

- Periodically evaluates and monitors the therapeutic response of the patient to prescribed drugs
- Reviews and interprets drug history to the physician, patient, or other persons involved with patient care
- Monitors patients' records for indications of drug abuse or misuse
- Reviews and/or seeks additional drug-related information (e.g., cost, pharmacokinetic characteristics, bioavailability, common adverse effect) to identify potential problems regarding drug therapy
- Reviews patient-related information for potential problems regarding drug therapy (e.g., socioeconomic factors, compliance habits, disease influences)
- Integrates drug-related with patient-related information to determine appropriate course of action (e.g., timing of dosage schedule, advising patient and/or other health professionals of possible adverse effects)
- Makes recommendations regarding drug therapy to the physician, patient, or other persons involved with patient's care

## Procedures

The pharmacist reviews the drug regimen of each patient at least monthly and reports any irregularities to the Medical Director, Director of Nursing Services, the attending physician, and the Administrator.

The term "drug regimen" or "medication regimen" means those drugs which are currently ordered for the patient and includes drugs which are on order but have not been recently used (PRNs).

The term "Irregularity" means failure to be in accord with what is usual, proper, accepted, or right.

Figure 4-2A
## MONTHLY MEDICATION SHEET

| MEDICATIONS | HOUR | 1 | 2 | 3 | 4 | 5 | 6 | 7 | 8 | 9 | 10 | 11 | 12 | 13 | 14 | 15 | 16 | 17 | 18 | 19 | 20 | 21 | 22 | 23 | 24 | 25 | 26 | 27 | 28 | 29 | 30 | 31 |
|---|---|---|---|---|---|---|---|---|---|---|---|---|---|---|---|---|---|---|---|---|---|---|---|---|---|---|---|---|---|---|---|---|

| Insulin Type | Hour Given | Amount Given | | | | | | | | | | | | | | | | | | | | | | | | | | | | | | | |
|---|---|---|---|---|---|---|---|---|---|---|---|---|---|---|---|---|---|---|---|---|---|---|---|---|---|---|---|---|---|---|---|---|---|
| | | Sugar | | | | | | | | | | | | | | | | | | | | | | | | | | | | | | | |
| | | Acetone | | | | | | | | | | | | | | | | | | | | | | | | | | | | | | | |

Site of Injection Code:  L.G. (Left Gluteus Muscle)   R.G. (Right Gluteus Muscle)   L.D. (Left Deltoid Muscle)   R.D. (Right Deltoid Muscle)
L.L. (Left Leg)   R.L. (Right Leg)   L.A. (Left Arm)   R.A. (Right Arm)

*Initial medication and identify initials below with signature*

| Nurses | Initial | Signature | Nurses | Initial | Signature | Nurses | Initial | Signature |
|---|---|---|---|---|---|---|---|---|
| A.M. Nurse | | | P.M. Nurse | | | Night Nurse | | |
| A.M. Relief | | | P.M. Relief | | | Relief Nurse | | |

| Last Name | First Name | Room No. | Patient No. | Date | Attending Physician |
|---|---|---|---|---|---|

**Figure 4-2B**
## MONTHLY PRN DRUG SHEET

| DATE | TIME | DRUG, DOSAGE, ROUTE, REASON | EFFECT | SIGNATURE |
|------|------|------------------------------|--------|-----------|
|      |      |                              |        |           |
|      |      |                              |        |           |
|      |      |                              |        |           |
|      |      |                              |        |           |
|      |      |                              |        |           |
|      |      |                              |        |           |
|      |      |                              |        |           |
|      |      |                              |        |           |
|      |      |                              |        |           |
|      |      |                              |        |           |
|      |      |                              |        |           |
|      |      |                              |        |           |
|      |      |                              |        |           |
|      |      |                              |        |           |
|      |      |                              |        |           |
|      |      |                              |        |           |
|      |      |                              |        |           |
|      |      |                              |        |           |
|      |      |                              |        |           |
|      |      |                              |        |           |
|      |      |                              |        |           |
|      |      |                              |        |           |
|      |      |                              |        |           |
|      |      |                              |        |           |
|      |      |                              |        |           |
|      |      |                              |        |           |
|      |      |                              |        |           |

| PATIENT NAME | PATIENT NO. | ROOM NO. | MO./YR. | PHYSICIAN | PAGE NO. |
|--------------|-------------|----------|---------|-----------|----------|

The pharmacist reviews each patient's drug regimen and associated factors in sufficient detail to determine if any irregularities exist. Irregularities may include drug-induced adverse reactions, interactions, duplicate therapy, and therapy no longer required. In performing the review, the pharmacist must have access to the patient, have an up-to-date record of all conditions the patient has which are likely to affect drug therapy, and have access to laboratory tests, physicians' progress notes, nurse's notes, and other documentation that will assist him or her in making a professional judgment whether or not irregularities exist in the drug regimen. Other documentation includes a monthly copy of the patient medication profile.

Each patient's drug regimen should be reviewed in the facility directly from the patient's medical record.

The pharmacist should provide the facility with documentation that he or she has reviewed each patient's drug regimen at least monthly. When possible irregularities are identified, the pharmacist should prepare a drug irregularity report and submit it to the medical director and the administrator. A follow-up report on each irregularity should be logged during the pharmacist's next visit to the facility. These reports should be stored and maintained in the facility on the same retention schedule as the patient's health records. The patient's drug regimen information form and reports should be maintained in the facility whether or not they are in the patient's chart. The pharmacist should not enter into the patient's health record statements that require or express medical judgment.

If the patient is interviewed, a separate list should be made indicating the criteria for the interview and listing the patients interviewed. This listing should be filed with the drug regimen review reports. The pharmacist should record a statement such as, "Drug therapy reviewed" to indicate that he or she has performed the review and sign and date the entry. This may be recorded in the section of the patient's health records marked "Physician Progress Notes." See sample Irregularity Report (Fig. 4-3), Drug Regimen Review and Report Form (Fig. 4-4), and Drug Regimen Review Profile Form (Fig. 4-5).

The Drug Regimen Review Profile Form is placed in a loose leaf notebook and kept in the facility. The form is designed to be used as a method of recording in brief:
- If the patient was interviewed and comments.
- If an Attention Required note was required and the follow-up action taken.
- If communication with the physician was required, the type of communication (phone, letter, in-person), and the follow-up action taken.

From time to time the pharmacist may want to make additional notations on this form in the space provided for pharmacist's progress notes.

Laboratory tests are monitored as well as various tests and studies for diabetes when appropriate.

Periodically (usually every 6 months), the number of medications ordered for the patient is recorded indicating how many are routine, PRN, and miscellaneous.

Effective performance of drug regimen review should result in improved therapy for the facility's patients and may lead to an overall cost savings. In many instances when comprehensive drug regimen review is initiated in a facility, a decrease in drug utilization will occur, as described in the review article "Saving Cost, Quality and People" that is included in the *Appendix*. More information and instructions on how to perform drug regimen reviews are available in the publication *Monitoring Drug Therapy in the Long-Term Care Facility* listed with the references at the end of this chapter.

# PARTICIPATION ON COMMITTEES

*Pharmacist's Responsibilities*

- Participates in utilization reviews, medical audits, and medical care evaluation and establishment of policies (e.g., as a member of medical care evaluation committee, peer review, pharmaceutical services committee, etc.)
- Assists in establishing, executing, tabulating, and evaluating clinical studies regarding drugs

Figure 4-3
**IRREGULARITY REPORT/DRUG REGIMEN REVIEW**

MONTH _____ FACILITY _____ STATION _____ TEAM _____

| ROOM NO. | ITEM NO. | PATIENT NAME | ACTION TAKEN |
|---|---|---|---|
|  |  |  |  |
|  |  |  |  |
|  |  |  |  |
|  |  |  |  |

PHARMACIST _____ PHARMD
INTERN/STUDENT _____

Carbon Copy:
Pharmacy
Administration
DNS

Figure 4-4
**PHARMACIST DRUG REGIMEN REVIEW AND REPORT**

ATTENTION REQUIRED

PATIENT _____
_____
_____
_____
_____

ACTION TAKEN: _____
_____

DATE _____ PHARMACIST _____
PHARMACY

## Drug Regimen Review and Report Form

One example of a pharmacist communication form is the four part carbonized Pharmacist Drug Regimen Review and Report. The first copy is perforated to give six individual tearout forms which are titled "Attention Required."

If the Pharmacist discovers an irregularity, the information is recorded on the Pharmacist Drug Regimen Review and Report form. The Attention Required slip is removed from the form and attached to the appropriate area in the patient's health records.

The Attention Required note clipped to the patient's health record is designed as a means of communicating the Pharmacist's findings to the various members of the staff including physicians.

In some cases action will be taken and in some cases no action will be taken. This action may be by a nurse, a physician or a pharmacist.

The action or non-action is indicated on the slip with the date of action and the slip is then forwarded to the Director of Nursing Services.

The Director of Nurses files the slip in the appropriate file with copies of the Pharmacist Drug Regimen Review and Reports.

# Procedures

The long-term care facility establishes committees to assure formal lines of communication among the personnel providing services offered to facility patients. These committees establish policies and procedures that govern the way services are provided. The pharmacist may be a member of the following committees: pharmaceutical services, infection control, utilization review, and patient care policy.

## Pharmaceutical Services Committee

The pharmaceutical services committee is usually composed of at least four persons: administrator, director of nursing service, pharmacist, and physician. Others on the committee might include the medical director, other physicians, and nurses.

The pharmaceutical services committee adopts and enforces policies and procedures concerning pharmaceutical service. The pharmacist carries out the policies and procedures established by this committee and reports to the committee on their use in the facility.

Figure 4-5A

## DRUG REGIMEN REVIEW PROFILE

PATIENT

AGE | WEIGHT

FACILITY | ALLERGIES:

PHYSICIAN

ROUTINE MEDICATIONS

PROBLEMS

| ADM. DATE | U.T.I. | D.M. | RESP./ARTH. | HYPTN./CHF | C.A.D./ARRYTH. | HEM. | G.I. | NEURO. | MISC. |
|---|---|---|---|---|---|---|---|---|---|

| NUMBER OF DRUGS | NUMBER OF DOSES PER DAY |
|---|---|
| ON ADD. | |
| ROUTINE | |
| PRN | |
| MISC. | |

| DATE | PATIENT INTERVIEW | COMMENTS | CONSULTANT PHARMACIST PHYSICIAN DRUG INFORMATION | RESPONSE | PHYSICIAN COMMUN- ICATION | RESPONSE | PHARMACIST COMMENTS |
|---|---|---|---|---|---|---|---|
| | | | | | | | |

The committee should meet at least quarterly and on the call of the chairman. The minutes of meetings should detail the committee's consideration of policies and procedures including recommendations for approval by the facility's patient care policy committee. The pharmaceutical services committee reviews reports submitted by the pharmacist and reports from official agency surveys. The committee takes appropriate action on recommendations contained in the reports and other suggestions that may be forthcoming from various members of the facility staff.

## Infection Control Committee

The infection control committee develops methods for investigating, controlling, and preventing infections in the facility. Members of this committee should include representatives from the medical, nursing, pharmacy, administrative, dietetic, housekeeping, and maintenance staff.

## Utilization Review Committee

The utilization review committee reviews all aspects of patient care to assure optimal utilization of all professional services. This committee evaluates admissions, length of patient stay, and appropriate use of professional material and services. Membership includes representatives of all health professions practicing in the facility. The pharmacist assesses drug and biological utilization in the facility.

## Patient Care Policy Committee

The patient care policy committee develops policies to govern skilled nursing care and related medical or other services the facility provides. The patient care policies should reflect provisions for meeting the total medical needs of patients, including admission, transfer, and discharge planning, and the range of services available to patients. These policies should include provisions to protect patients' personal and property rights. The members of this committee should include one or more physicians and registered nurses, the pharmacist, and administrator.

# INSERVICE EDUCATION

*Pharmacist's Responsibilities*

- Provides drug information to other health care professionals in a formal setting (e.g., organizes inservice educational programs, lectures, seminars, exhibits)
- Organizes or participates in "in pharmacy" education programs for other pharmacists
- Instructs and trains pharmacists and nonpharmacist staff in carrying out their assigned responsibilities
- Selects, evaluates, organizes, and maintains a current library of drug information for use of pharmacy and facility personnel in their training and conduct of their day-to-day operation

## Procedures

The pharmacist is generally expected to participate in ongoing inservice training for facility staff regularly. The administrator, director of nursing service, or physicians on the staff may request specialized lectures or discussions in the area of drugs as needs arise.

The pharmacist may provide bulletin board material and other reference material and resources for continuing education of facility personnel. A continual review and updating of federal, state, and local laws and regulations as they apply to the long-term care facility should be included in the inservice programs. Various teaching techniques should be used to provide interesting and informative programs, such as visual aids, quizzes, lectures, written outlines, and group discussion. A record of each inservice program must be maintained listing the topic and names of those present.

## Reference Materials

The facility should maintain reference materials containing drug monographs on all drugs in use in the facility as well as current drug reference texts and sources of information. Such monographs must include information concerning generic and brand names, if applicable; available strengths and dosage forms; and pharmacological data including indications and side effects. These reference texts should be accessible at all times to the professional staff of the facility so that no drug is administered unless information on actions, side effects, and contraindications is available on the floor of the nursing unit. Some examples of appropriate texts are the *Evaluations of Drug Interactions, Handbook of Nonprescription Drugs, The American Hospital Formulary Service, Facts and Comparisons, The Merck Manual, American Medical Association Drug Evaluations*, manufacturers information such as the *Physicians' Desk Reference* or package inserts, a medical dictionary, and a pharmacology text. A current copy of the facility's formulary (if there is a formulary) should be available at each nursing station also. The pharmacy must have any texts required by law, such as the USP.

# PATIENT DISCHARGE COUNSELING

*Pharmacist's Responsibilities*

- Advises patients or responsible party of potential drug- and health-related conditions that may develop from the use of medication for which the patient should seek other medical care
- Confirms and further clarifies patient's understanding of medication dosage, dosage frequency, and method of administration
- Consults with patient to identify properly symptoms to advise patient for self-medication
- Refers patient to other health care providers and/or health resources where indicated
- Advises patients on personal health matters (e.g., smoking or drug abuse)

## Procedures

There may be instances in which long-term care patients are discharged to their home or other self-care environment from the long-term care facility. When this occurs, the pharmacist should be involved in teaching the patient about proper adherence to the drug therapy. Studies have shown that careful instruction in their drug therapy before discharge increases the likelihood of patients' compliance with therapy. Instruction may include information about time, route, frequency of drug administration, and any other information pertinent to patient care. Compliance aids might also be provided.

## References for Further Reading

Baxendale, C. *et al.*, "A Self-Medication Retraining Program," *Br. Med. J., 2*, 1278(1978).

Brown, C. H., "Committee Involvement by Consultant Pharmacists in Extended Care Facilities," *Indiana Pharm., 58*, 170(July 1977).

Kabat, H. F. *et al., Drug Utilization Review in Skilled Nursing Facilities*, Department of Health, Education, and Welfare, Public Health Service, November 1975.

Kalman, S. H., *Monitoring Drug Therapy in the Long-Term Care Facility*, American Pharmaceutical Association, Washington, D.C., 1978.

Kalman, S. H., *The Right Drug to the Right Patient*, American Pharmaceutical Association, Washington, D.C., 1977.

Kidder, S. W., "Saving Cost, Quality and People: Drug Reviews in Long-Term Care," *Am. Pharm., NS18*, 346(1978).

Lipman, A. G., "Drug Dosage Consideration in Elderly Patients," *Modern Medicine, 8*, 87(April 30, 1978).

Stewart, J. E. *et al.*, "Monitoring Drug Therapy in Skilled Nursing Facility Patients," *Drug Intell. Clin. Pharm., 12*, 704(1978).

Wartak, J. and T. Bryce Miller, "Decision Tables for Planning Drug Therapy," *Drug Intell. Clin. Pharm., 13*, 100(1979).

**Figure 4-5B**

| PROGRESS NOTES | DPH LEVEL (10-20 mcg/ml) | INSULIN |
|---|---|---|
| | Ph LEVEL (10-45 mcg/ml) | ORAL |
| | QUINIDINE LEVEL (2-5 mcg/ml) | DIET |

| | | | | | | | | | | | | |
|---|---|---|---|---|---|---|---|---|---|---|---|---|
| DATE | | | | | | | | | | | | |
| U/A: | | | | | | | | | | | | |
| S.G. (1.010-1.030) | | | | | | | | | | | | |
| pH (5-8) | | | | | | | | | | | | |
| PROTEIN (None-Min.amt.) | | | | | | | | | | | | |
| WBC/hpf (None) | | | | | | | | | | | | |
| RBC/hpf (None) | | | | | | | | | | | | |
| CASTS (None) | | | | | | | | | | | | |
| GLUCOSE (None) | | | | | | | | | | | | |
| ACETONE (None) | | | | | | | | | | | | |
| BACT. | | | | | | | | | | | | |
| C/S: | | | | | | | | | | | | |
| LAB STUDIES | | | | | | | | | | | | |
| FBS 70-110 mg% | | | | | | | | | | | | |
| S/A | | | | | | | | | | | | |
| HGB/HCT 11-17/37-54 | | | | | | | | | | | | |
| MCV | | | | | | | | | | | | |
| MCH | | | | | | | | | | | | |
| MCHC | | | | | | | | | | | | |
| WBC | | | | | | | | | | | | |
| PLATELETS | | | | | | | | | | | | |

| | | | | | | | | | | | | |
|---|---|---|---|---|---|---|---|---|---|---|---|---|
| LAB STUDIES | | | | | | | | | | | | |
| BUN/CR | | | | | | | | | | | | |
| DIG. LEVEL 0.9-2.0 ng/ml | | | | | | | | | | | | |
| Na/K (136-145/3.5-5.0 mEq/L) | | | | | | | | | | | | |
| Cl/$CO_2$ (96-106/25-31 MEq/L) | | | | | | | | | | | | |
| URIC ACID 3-8 mg% | | | | | | | | | | | | |

# Chapter 5:
# PLANNING

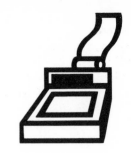

The first step on the road to providing pharmaceutical services to long-term care facilities is planning. Planning includes:
- Assessing opportunities and facility characteristics
- Designing the pharmaceutical service package
- Analyzing the financial and economic picture
- Preparing a written plan of implementation.

A good plan helps you anticipate exactly what will occur at each step of establishing and providing services. The purpose of the plan is to minimize surprises. Ninety percent of the effort that goes into any successful project occurs during the planning phase. This chapter suggests some factors to consider in preparing your plan. The lists, forms, and questions are designed to help you think through what you need to know and do. Your chances for success are better if you understand the problems you will meet and work out as many of them as you can before you start.

## ASSESSING THE OPPORTUNITIES AND FACILITY CHARACTERISTICS

Planning means making many decisions before taking action. A basic decision you will make at this point is whether you want to serve long-term care facilities or not. If you are going to serve LTCFs, you should decide in a very systematic fashion what services you will—or can—provide and how. This decision should be based on your desires and ability to provide service and the facility's needs and wants. To make this decision, you will necessarily perform a balancing act to derive a desirable mix of economically feasible services. The planning process allows you time to determine what is realistic and what will satisfy the many interests that regulate long-term care to avoid misunderstandings or worse problems later. Careful *self-assessment*, combined with your *assessment of the needs of the long-term care facility* in question, is required.

Pharmaceutical services are divided into dispensing and nondispensing services. Dispensing services mean those functions directly connected to dispensing prescriptions, such as interpreting the order, labeling and packaging the drug, and delivery. Nondispensing services include clinical and administrative tasks not directly associated with dispensing, such as inservice education, drug administration, and drug regimen review. These concepts and services are discussed fully in Chapter 2. Figure 2-1 illustrates the sequence of activities involved in serving long-term care patients. If you are uncertain about the distinction between the two types of services, refer to Chapter 2 before continuing with planning.

## WHAT ARE THE NEEDS OF LONG-TERM CARE FACILITIES?

Long-term care facility's needs for service are determined in part by legal and regulatory requirements and also by unique characteristics of the facility. State, federal, and local laws and regulations and voluntary standards affect long-term care. These effects are discussed in detail in Chapters 1-4. Generally, laws, regulations, and voluntary standards dictate some services that LTCFs *must provide* for their residents. The standards may also specify *how* services are to be performed along with criteria for evaluating the quality of service. The *Appendix* contains copies of the federal regulations. You can obtain copies of applicable state laws and regulations from your state health and/or welfare department, state board of pharmacy, and/or state pharmaceutical association. The facility may be voluntarily accredited by the Joint Commission on the Accreditation of Hospitals (JCAH). The *Appendix* also contains a copy of the JCAH standards. You must have a detailed understanding of present and possible future requirements before investing substantial effort beyond just thinking about serving LTCFs.

If the facility does not participate in Medicare or Medicaid, only state or local licensure laws apply. In some states, the requirements for a LTCF license are less stringent than the federal regulations. However, if the facility decides to participate in Medicare and Medicaid, it must meet the federal requirements. Such a change while you are providing service would mean a revision in the service needs and is obviously something to investigate. If you are aware of the all possible legal and voluntary standards, especially when change is anticipated, you can prepare for them. Regulations are revised periodically. You should stay informed of changes in these external factors that can directly affect your service.

These requirements delineate the basic set of services LTCFs need. However, you must also decide what services and methods of provision accommodate the facility's unique needs. The information you gather is taken from the facility's past experience, its present system, and its projected future requirements.

## Long-Term Care Facility Vital Statistics

In Chapter 1, the unique characteristics of each facility were divided into four categories: physical, ownership, staff, and patient. A detailed list of data on each characteristic can help in your planning. The Long-Term Care Facility Vital Statistics Form in Planning Worksheet #1 is one device for collecting necessary information conveniently. Most information on this form can and should be gathered before you begin formal discussions with the facility administrator. Sources of information include state and local nursing home associations, state licensing and accrediting bodies, and printed materials distributed by the facility. Any information you are unable to collect ahead of time can be obtained from the administrator, director of nursing, medical director, and other staff.

Collection of this information systematically helps you to:
- determine service needs, potential costs, and tasks to be completed before implementation
- make a comparative evaluation of facilities
- impress the administrator with your thoroughness in doing a job
- define areas of possible future development
- estimate expected compensation

The form begins with routine information to identify the facility: its name, address, telephone number, and the names of the individuals in key administrative positions, the administrator, director of nursing, and medical director.

Physical and ownership characteristics are included in the section titled "Facility Data." The first item is ownership. The facility owners have the final authority on policies; they handle financial aspects of the operation; and they make the contracts for services. By identifying ownership, you also identify the important decision makers—the individuals you ultimately will have to convince to be successful. The facility accreditation and certification tell you which standards, other than those mandated in the state licensure laws, the facility must meet. It can also indicate to some extent the quality of care provided. The facility size affects how much equipment and other resources will be needed and whether special equipment will be necessary to suit any physical idiosyncracies of the building.

If there is a pharmacy on-premises, you must determine if the size is adequate for the number of beds. Once you have made a final decision on what will be provided, it will be necessary to reassess any on-premises pharmacy to determine whether it is still adequate.

The location of an off-premises pharmacy in relation to the facility is important in determining drug delivery needs. An off-premises pharmacy that provides dispensing services obviously must have a delivery service to transport drugs from the pharmacy to the facility. The relative location of the facility directly affects the time required and the amount of fuel

# Planning Worksheet #1

## Long-Term Care Facility Vital Statistics

NAME OF FACILITY _____ ADMINISTRATOR _____

ADDRESS _____ DIRECTOR OF NURSING _____

TELEPHONE _____ MEDICAL DIRECTOR _____

### FACILITY DATA

Facility Ownership _____

Facility Accreditation and Certification

    JCAH _____

    Medicare _____

    Medicaid _____

Number of Beds _____

Number of Nursing Units _____

Storage of Drugs at Nursing Units

    Size of Space _____

    Type of Space _____
    (e.g. cabinets, carts, etc.)

Arrangements for transporting drugs in the Facility (e.g. elevators, stairs)

_____

For on-premises pharmacy:

Size of Pharmacy _____

Location of Pharmacy in Facility _____

_____

For off-premises pharmacy:

Distance of Facility From Pharmacy _____

_____

### PATIENT DATA

#### Number of Patients According to Level of Care and Payment Source

| Payment Source / Level of Care | SNF | ICF | OTHER | TOTAL |
|---|---|---|---|---|
| Medicaid | | | | |
| Medicare | | XXXX | XXXX | |
| Other 3rd Parties | XXXX | XXXX | | |
| Private | XXXX | XXXX | | |
| TOTAL | | | | |

Average New Admissions
Per Month _____

Average Discharges
Per Month _____

Average Length of Stay _____

Average Number of Prescriptions Per Patient Per Month _____

### STAFF DATA

Number of Nurses _____

Other staff _____

_____

_____

Number of Physicians _____

_____

_____

### COMMENTS

_____

_____

_____

necessary. All of these factors affect the time, resources, and costs of providing service.

The "Patient Data" section breaks down the number and type of patients by level of care and payment source. The level of care may indicate the amount and type of drugs patients will be taking. Patients requiring a higher level of care are likely to receive more drugs. The payment source combined with the level of care stipulates the compensation that you can expect from third-party programs. For example, some state Medicaid programs have established different fee levels for skilled nursing and intermediate care facility patients. Because individual prescription fees are established by the state financing agency, the compensation for serving Medicaid recipients can be ascertained easily by checking with the state Medicaid agency on current fee levels.

Admissions and discharges represent sources of cost in the system. Each time a patient is admitted or discharged there are added administrative costs to delete his or her records and supplies in the medication system.

The number of prescriptions per patient per unit time multiplied by the average number of patients yields an estimate of the prescription volume. For instance, a 100-bed facility with a monthly average of six prescriptions per patient would require 600 prescriptions per month. If the pharmacy dispenses 5 days per week (or 20 days per month), this facility would generate about 30 prescriptions per day. Obviously, there are factors that will cause the daily—and even the monthly—averages to fluctuate. As a planning tool, you should estimate what the situation would be with a $\pm 10\%$ variation or preferably the actual variation of the facility in question.

If you intend to provide dispensing services, the prescription volume is essential to estimate your resource requirements. If you base compensation on a per prescription fee, this figure alone specifies, to a large extent, the total compensation for dispensing services. If the patient turnover is high, however, there may be a great deal of fluctuation in the prescription volume. New admissions may receive drastically different quantities of drugs than the patients discharged; therefore frequent changes in the patient population can affect the prescription volume.

One way to collect more specific information about drug utilization is to review the charts of every patient in the facility before preparing a service proposal. You may record every drug taken, the approximate frequency of use (i.e., number of doses per day), and whether regularly scheduled or PRN. As a by-product of this activity, you can estimate the drug usage and initial inventory requirements with a high degree of precision. In addition, this survey may serve as an initial drug regimen review—a baseline measure of how well or poor present services meet patient needs and how much effort will be required on your part to bring all services to an acceptable level.

The staff data focus on nurses and physicians. When compared with data from other facilities, this information should help you to determine whether staffing is adequate, the amount of personnel turnover, and the nature of staff interactions. Staff data may reveal another source of potential service costs. For example, if the staff turnover is high, frequent inservice training sessions may be necessary to acquaint staff with drug distribution system procedures. High employee turnover also delays service and adds to your costs by requiring more calls, more trips to the facility, and more intensive monitoring of the delivery process.

Some information and discussion about costs and service data may seem obvious or simple to you; however, gathering these data systematically helps you compare various facilities and build a data base to detect sources of potential problems *before* you decide to serve a facility. By planning, you may be able to eliminate some problems and be ready for those that do occur.

## Service, Personnel, and Cost Interactions

Table 5-1 lists the facility characteristics that affect personnel needs, labor, and equipment costs for each service activity. Although it is not possible to assign absolute numbers to these factors, comparative information for several facilities should allow an assessment of relative service costs and needs.

Table 5-1

# HOW THE FACILITY'S VITAL STATISTICS AFFECT
# THE COST OF PROVIDING SERVICE

| Service Component | Facility Characteristic | Affects Personnel Requirements | Affects Labor Costs | Affects Equipment Costs |
|---|---|---|---|---|
| **DISPENSING SERVICES** | | | | |
| 1. Medication Order | Number of orders<br>Number of physicians<br>Distance of pharmacy<br>  from facility | RPh &<br>nonRPh | Time required to<br>  receive, review<br>  and verify orders | Forms<br>Telephone<br>Telecopier<br>Photocopier |
| 2. Patient Medication Profile | Number of patients<br>Number of orders | RPh | Time to review and<br>  fill information | Forms<br>Storage and retrieval<br>  systems space |
| 3. Dispensing | Number of prescriptions<br>Distribution system | RPh &<br>nonRPh | Time to package,<br>  label, etc. | Packaging materials<br>equipment, labels |
| 4. Delivery | Distance of pharmacy<br>  from facility<br>Transportation to and<br>  inside facility | RPh &<br>nonRPh | Time to transport,<br>  administrative<br>  time | Car or truck<br>Special transport<br>  equipment |
| 5. Storage | Number of patients<br>Number of prescriptions<br>Size of pharmacy<br>Storage in facility<br>Type of storage | RPh &<br>nonRPh | Checking for out-<br>  dated drugs<br>Monitoring storage | Space in pharmacy &<br>  LTCF<br>Special containers<br>Security systems<br>Forms |
| 6. Accountability | Size of facility<br>Size of staff | RPh | Time to keep and<br>  review records | Forms |
| **NONDISPENSING SERVICES** | | | | |
| 1. Administration | Number of nursing<br>  units<br>Number of patients | NonRPh | Nursing time | Forms, Kardex, MAR<br>Cups, syringes, needles |
| 2. Drug Regimen Review | Number of patients<br>Number of prescriptions<br>Number of nurses &<br>  physicians<br>Levels of care | RPh | Time (may be<br>  determined per<br>  patient) | Forms, travel,<br>  communication<br>  devices |
| 3. Committees | Size of facility | RPh | Preparation and<br>  attendance time | Forms |
| 4. Inservice Education | Size of staff | RPh | Preparation and<br>  attendance | Teaching equipment,<br>  supplies, books,<br>  AV aids |
| 5. Patient Discharge Counseling | Number of discharges | RPh | Time to counsel | Education tools |

The costs associated with each service activity are divided into labor and equipment. Personnel requirements are listed as pharmacists and nonpharmacists. Nonpharmacists may include pharmacy supportive personnel, nurses, nurses' aides, or other individuals associated with the medication system. The facility characteristics are taken from the Long-Term Care Facility Vital Statistics form. For example, the number of orders, number of physicians, and distance of the pharmacy from the facility affect the resource requirements associated with the medication order. The pharmacy personnel requirements and costs that are affected include pharmacists' time required to receive, review, and verify orders and the cost of forms, telephone, and telecopier or photocopier to duplicate the original orders. Nurses and pharmacy aides may also be involved in transmitting orders. In general, a larger or more complex characteristic of the facility implies a higher pharmacy cost. The section on economic considerations describes methods of defining costs. The purpose of Table 5-1 is to assist in listing and categorizing all sources of service costs and relating them to facility characteristics. A review of this table shows you how each activity is affected by the facility's characteristics.

## Critical Subjective Factors

Besides the "quantitative" characteristics of the facility that affect service, such as number of patients and number of prescriptions, there are facility traits that you should assess subjectively. Look at the overall organization of services as well as each characteristic. For example, not only is the number of orders significant but the system for transmitting orders is equally important. If the facility ordering system is disorganized, there may be a disproportionately high frequency of emergency orders and night calls. If staff interrelationships are poor, lack of cooperation may undermine even the best planned and theoretically efficient system.

The following questions concern the critical factors needed to assess these subjective traits.

- Why is the facility seeking a new pharmaceutical services provider?
    Is it a new facility?
    Was the previous provider unsatisfactory to the facility?
    Was the previous provider dissatisfied with the facility?
- Are any changes in the facility's characteristics planned in the future?
    Will the facility be expanding?
    Will the facility's system or organization be changing?
    Does the facility plan to add or drop services?
    Do different staff members have the same view of future directions for the facility?
- Are changes in management or ownership of the facility likely in the near future?
    How old is management?
    How long have they worked at this facility?
- Is the facility financially sound?
    Does it pay its suppliers on time?
    Does it pay its employees on time?
    Has the Better Business Bureau received complaints about it?
- What changes or improvements are needed in the facility's operation?
    What do different staff members think are the facility's biggest problems?
    What do different staff members think are the facility's greatest assets?
    What are the attitudes of staff members toward each other?
    How does the turnover of staff compare with other facilities?
- Do you have a favorable impression of the facility overall?

The administrator, director of nursing, medical director, other staff, and any pharmacists who have previously served the facility are the most likely sources of answers. This list is not exhaustive. Add or change questions for any additional factors that you feel are needed. If your responses to these questions give an unfavorable picture, you may not want to serve the facility or it may represent a challenge. Even if the picture is favorable, you still may lack the desire or capability to serve it. You must assess your own needs and wants.

# DESIGNING THE PHARMACEUTICAL SERVICE PACKAGE

To begin your self-assessment, look at your personal strengths and weaknesses. Ask yourself a few general questions if this is your first venture into managing and offering your services. Even if you currently are the owner or manager of a pharmacy you may wish to evaluate how a change of operation will affect you personally. The Small Business Administration suggests the following questions:

- Are you a self-starter?
- Do you get along with other people?
- Can you lead others?
- Can you take responsibility?
- Are you a good organizer?
- Are you a good worker?
- Can you make decisions?
- Can people trust what you say?
- Can you stick with it?
- Is your health good?

Besides these general questions, look at the nature of providing service to long-term care facilities:

- Do you have experience serving long-term care facilities?
- Do you understand the needs of long-term care patients?
- Are you familiar with the drug therapy of the common diseases of long-term care patients?
- Do you understand the organizational system of long-term care facilities?
- Can you provide emergency services during off-hours?
- Can you work on institutional committees?
- Do you have the equipment, supplies, and other resources needed? If not, can you afford and finance them?

As mentioned in Chapter 2, you may choose to provide all or a portion of the set of services needed by the facility. For example, some pharmacists provide only the dispensing services and others only nondispensing services. Several examples were described in Chapter 2. Whether you can find facilities needing only select services depends on your area. Some facilities prefer to obtain all of their pharmaceutical services from one provider, while others diversify because of advantages that different providers offer. Some pharmacists, who want to offer comprehensive services but do not have the resources, subcontract with other pharmacists for a portion of the services. The flexibility in the range of services you may choose to provide is limited primarily by what your colleagues are willing to do and the demand for services in your area.

At this point, you may wish to list the services you plan to provide (see Chapters 2–4 and Table 5-2). Next prepare a list of the equipment, supplies, and other resources that you have and need. Table 5-2 lists each service component and the resources required for each. Dispensing activities obviously require pharmacy space, dispensing equipment, record keeping supplies, and pharmacists' and nonpharmacists' time. Nondispensing activities require supplies and pharmacists' time both in direct provision of service and preparation through education and report writing. Planning Worksheet #2 offers one method of organizing your services and resource needs. All services are listed in the first column. The resource requirements, as indicated on the worksheet, should be divided into those on-hand and those that must be acquired. You may prepare a general summary list first and then look at each resource further to ferret out all potential costs and necessary activities. For example, if you have a pharmacy, it may require remodeling. There are maintenance, rent, and depreciation factors to consider. Figure 5-1 summarizes how a list might look for dispensing services. The cost estimates in columns 4, 5, and 6 are discussed in the next section.

Table 5-2

# PHARMACIST'S PLANNING LIST

| *Service Component* | *Pharmacist's Required Resources* |
|---|---|
| **DISPENSING SERVICES** | Must have a licensed pharmacy either on facility's premises or off-premises |
| 1. Receipt of Medication Order | Must have a means of obtaining order from facility—via telephone—and also written copies of orders |
| 2. Maintenance of Patient Medication Profile | Must have system of patient medication profiles for all patients in a facility. Requires storage space. Should be segregated from records of outpatients and other facilities' patients. |
| 3. Labeling and Dispensing the Drug Order | Must have adequate personnel and space to perform, regardless of the distribution system. May require special packaging and labeling equipment, depending on distribution system. |
| 4. Delivery of Drugs | An off-premises pharmacy must have routine delivery service, and a means of supplying stat and emergency drugs. An on-premises pharmacy must transport drugs to nursing units. May require special carts, depending on distribution system. |
| 5. Storage | Requires adequate space in pharmacy and in facility for necessary inventory, records, and equipment, including workspace. |
| 6. Accountability | Must keep medication records from point of medication order to administration or disposition of drugs supplied to the facility. |
| **NONDISPENSING SERVICES** | |
| 1. Administration of Drugs | Must be familiar with procedures in order to compile policy and procedure manual. |
| 2. Review of Drug Regimen | Requires traveling to facility, reviewing each patient's records (usually monthly), following up findings. Must have drug knowledge expertise. |
| 3. Participation on Committees | Requires preparation time, attendance at meetings and follow-up. |
| 4. Inservice Education | Requires preparation and attendance, as well as teaching aids. |
| 5. Patient Discharge Counseling | Requires preparation time and time to perform. May need teaching and compliance aids. |

## Analyzing The Economic Picture

The costs associated with providing services can be divided into start-up and sustaining costs. Start-up costs are one-time costs that occur when a new service is initiated. They can be further subdivided into asset investment and initial operating costs.

In Fig. 5-1, for example, the planning list indicates that the pharmacist would need to remodel the pharmacy, purchase additional equipment, and add to the pharmacy's inventory. All of these costs are listed in the "initial cost" column. They are considered asset investments because they increase the investment level of the pharmacy and are reflected on the balance sheet.

## Planning Worksheet #2

**REQUIRED RESOURCES**

Page _____ of _____

Facility Name _____     Number of Beds _____

| Service Component | Required Personnel, Equipment, and Supplies | | Total Cost Estimate | | |
|---|---|---|---|---|---|
| | On-hand | Must Acquire | Initial | Monthly | Yearly or Quarterly |
| 1 | 2 | 3 | 4 | 5 | 6 |
| | | | | | |
| | | | | | |
| | | | | | |
| | | | | | |
| | | | | | |
| | | | | | |
| | | | | | |
| | | | | | |
| | | | | | |
| | | | | | |
| | | | | | |
| | | | | | |
| | | | | | |
| | | | | | |
| | | | | | |
| | | | | | |
| | | | | | |
| | | | | | |
| | | | | | |
| | | | | | |
| | | | | | |
| | | | | | |

Figure 5-1*
Sample
**Planning Worksheet #2**

REQUIRED RESOURCES

Facility Name _General NH_     Number of Beds _100_

| Service Component | Required Personnel, Equipment, and Supplies | | Total Cost Estimate *(during first year of operation)* | | |
|---|---|---|---|---|---|
| | On-hand | Must Acquire | Initial | Monthly | Yearly or Quarterly |
| 1 | 2 | 3 | 4 | 5 | 6 |
| Dispensing Services Lease of | off premises pharmacy | contractor estimate for remodeling | 1910.00 | | |
| Medication Order | telephone | (add a line) Install | 52.00 | 12.00 | |
| | | 6 dozen order forms @ 4.30 each | 345.60 | → | one year supply |
| | Photocopier | 600 copies at 5¢ each | | 30.00 | |
| Patient Profile | profile system | one additional storage bin | 22.50 | | |
| Dispensing | labels, | one box per month | | 15.00 | |
| | unit dose pack- machine | delivery & install tax added below | 450.00 | | |
| | Record forms | 200 forms for one year | 100.00 | → | one year supply |
| (6 Rx/Pt/Mo → total *36.00 life cost) assume 2 turns - avg inven. 1st yr | | additional inventory | 4500.00 | | |
| | unit dose pack supplies | 600 doses/month @ plega | $12.00×12mo | 12.00 | |
| | technician | 40 hrs/week (3.20 + 0.45/hr) | | 319.00 | |
| | pharmacist | 40 hrs/week (10 + 1.50 per hr) | | 1994.00 | |
| Delivery | (truck - already own) | | | | |
| | driver | 20 hrs/week (3.20 + 0.45/hr) | | 319.00 | |
| | fuel, maintenance, etc | | | 40.00 | |
| Storage | | $450/cart 5 carts for facility | 2400.00 | | |
| Accountability | | schI & cs forms | 45.00 | → | one year supply |
| | | inventory forms | | | |
| Miscellaneous - Billing/Bookkeeping | | 2 hrs/wk plus 10 hrs/mo | | 374.00 | |
| | | finance 3 months accts receivable | 13,600.00 | | |
| Sales Tax - 5% taxable items | | | 177.00 | 2.35 | |
| Total for Phase one | | | 23,626.10 | 3118.35 | |

*The figures in this example are reasonable, but hypothetical. They are used merely to illustrate the planning process.

Operating capital is the initial amount of cash needed to finance operations until payments on accounts begin to be collected. For example, the pharmacy must purchase forms, supplies, and drugs to begin operating but will not begin to collect accounts receivable until the second or third month of operation. Therefore, the costs of these initial purchases must be financed with operating funds. The initial costs for items that are not asset investments represent increases in required operating capital and include such things as supplies and at least 2 months provision of wages, payroll taxes, and benefits for personnel and other initial operating costs listed in Fig. 5-1.

Sustaining costs are the ongoing costs of operating the pharmacy and providing service. In Fig. 5-1, these include the costs listed in columns 5 and 6. Sustaining costs are usually made up of direct and indirect costs.

Direct costs can be associated readily and easily with a particular operating department or operation of the pharmacy, such as prescription dispensing.[1] Indirect or common costs cannot be readily identified with a particular operating department. Direct cost items listed in Fig. 5-1 include unit dose packaging equipment, forms, and supplies associated with serving the LTCF, and that portion of the wages of each employee that covers their time in dispensing LTCF prescriptions.

Indirect costs include such costs as rent and utilities associated with housing the pharmacy, costs associated with general management, and costs from delivery that cannot be directly assigned to the delivery of prescriptions to the facility. Only the costs that can be allocated without question to the LTCF operating department should be listed.

For an on-premises pharmacy, which serves only the facility in which it is located, *all* costs may be assigned to an overall pharmacy operating department. For pharmacies serving more than one facility and/or out-patients in addition to LTCF service, costs should be allocated to the specific LTCF service operating department.

Among the many procedures for allocating indirect costs, the most frequently used methods involve the use of physical measures or revenue amounts. The methods based on physical measures utilize some physical attribute common to all indirect costs to allocate costs to the LTCF operating department. Floor space, weight, and volume are frequently used. Under this procedure, the common cost is allocated on the basis of each department's relative proportion of the physical measure, such as percent of floor space.

Another common method of allocating indirect costs is the revenue percentage method. Costs, using this method, are allocated to each department proportionately according to its revenue. For example, advertising can be allocated to the prescription operating department based on the proportion of prescription revenue to total revenue.

A less frequently used method is to allocate costs on the benefits received. This method might be appropriate for allocating central office administrative expenses and possibly for nondispensing service costs. These expenses could be allocated in the amount of time expended and number of reports developed by the pharmacy.

Lastly, expenses can be allocated by other less common methods or a combination of methods. APhA's *Uniform Cost Accounting System* contains more detailed information on cost allocation. You should consult your accounting advisor on these matters, because inappropriate assessment of costs is a leading cause of failure in a new endeavor.

Direct and indirect costs can be either fixed or variable. Fixed costs do not change regardless of fluctuations in volume of activity. Variable costs fluctuate directly with revenue or other measured activities, such as prescription volume, number of beds, or amount of time spent providing service. For the purposes of listing the variable costs in columns 5 and 6 of Worksheet #2, you may either list the cost for a defined variable, such as the 100 beds used in the example (Fig. 5-1), or you may list the total cost per unit, such as the cost per bed or per prescription.

The total of the initial costs from column 4 tells you how much cash, equity, and credit you will need to begin operation. These are also called "sunk" costs—costs that will have to be committed to the activity to begin offering a service. The information in columns 5 and 6 is used to assist you in evaluating cost recovery (discussed later in this chapter).

# Listing Costs

The numbers in Figure 5-1 are fictitious figures to illustrate how the form is filled out. There are many sources of information about specific costs that you can apply to your own situation. The *Appendix* contains an extensive list of manufacturers and suppliers of equipment for pharmaceutical service to long-term care facilities. State and national pharmaceutical journals, professional associations, and state boards of pharmacy also have information. Professional association annual meeting exhibits offer access to many manufacturers' representatives in one location for information on specific products.

In addition to APhA's Academy of Pharmacy Practice Section on Long Term Care, many of the state pharmaceutical associations have long-term care groups. If you are interested in a particular product or system, you might contact colleagues who use the system, to see it in operation and learn about their professional and personal experiences. The Small Business Administration has many helpful booklets and many universities have small business institutes that provide consultation. When shopping around for the equipment and services you will need, obtain written competitive bids where possible. Make sure that each bid specifies how long the offer is binding, for example, how long the supplier will guarantee the price.

A major portion of the expenses that you identify are essential and cannot be avoided. There may be methods of minimizing expenses in some areas and timing to avoid expenses at a difficult period. However, failure to identify expenses in the planning phase can lead to disaster later. Return to your list of expenses once again and search for all possible sources of costs. You will generally find that from 50 to 80% of these costs are fixed.

Keep in mind that there may be hidden costs "behind" the item you have written on your list. For example, "behind" your estimates for wages and salaries are payroll taxes (FICA, workers compensation, unemployment compensation, and local payroll taxes) and benefits. The total salary expense is generally 1.20 to 1.40 times the nominal salary. If your planning is considerably ahead of implementing service, include an inflation factor. For equipment costs, be sure to include sales tax, shipping, installation, and delivery charges where applicable. If you must borrow money, include the cost of credit. When you have listed all of the costs, total them, and add 10 to 20% contingency to the total to allow a cushion for error.

# Financing Costs

The initial investment might be financed using your personal funds, shifting capital away from a pre-existing operation and by borrowing capital. If you plan to borrow, it is wise to begin early to develop a relationship with the lender to obtain favorable rates. In some cases, it may be beneficial to borrow the money shortly before it is needed if interest rates are better at that time. Before borrowing you should develop a cash flow budget to show how the loan will be repaid. An accountant or financial adviser may be helpful.

Other sources of credit include suppliers to the pharmacy or a line of credit arrangement with a bank. A line of credit can be used to fund seasonal fluctuations and to cushion against any underestimation in accounts receivable.

# Reducing Costs

Although most costs are fixed and often unavoidable, there are strategies to modify your cost pattern.
- Lease your equipment or arrange to share it with another pharmacy.
- Use a courier service instead of buying a delivery vehicle and hiring a driver.
- Hire part-time help at first.
- Modularize your service package in order to implement it in steps.
- Use pharmacy aides when possible.
- Train nursing staff to coordinate ordering.
- Accelerate depreciation to reduce taxation.

- Share product purchasing with another pharmacy to benefit from quantity discounts or direct purchasing.
- Minimize inventory by arranging to purchase infrequently prescribed drugs from another pharmacy.
- Arrange financing with a wholesaler to start-up inventory.
- Buy on consignment and utilize "datings" so that you are working on your supplier's money.
- Arrange financing with suppliers of equipment.
- Monitor returns to the pharmacy and implement policies to reduce returns.
- Call ahead before going to meetings.
- Use nursing home personnel as technicians in the pharmacy—for an on-premises pharmacy.
- Offer employees compensatory time for off-hours service and cut down on excess staffing during the day.
- Stipulate in the contract with the facility the number of emergency calls to be covered and tier the fee structure for excess calls.

All of these suggestions involve assessing the situation and looking for any possible sources of efficiency.

## Recovering Costs

Cost recovery can be projected by budgeting, performing a break-even analysis, and constructing a cash flow projection. A budget is a detailed plan of future expenditures and receipts. By completing Worksheet #2, you have begun to prepare a budget. From Worksheet #2 you can directly determine the start-up costs required to initiate service. The next step in budgeting is to project the profit or loss expected once service is initiated. One management aid to help accomplish this is a break-even analysis.

The break-even point is the point at which the pharmacy's total revenues equal the total expenses. Aggregate costs must be recovered in order to break-even. The costs listed in columns 5 and 6 of Worksheet #2 can be used to conduct a break-even analysis. In addition, the start-up or sunk costs can be included by using an amortization or depreciation schedule. A detailed discussion of amortization is beyond the scope of this book. For more information, see the Internal Revenue Service tax guide and consult your accountant.

The costs for a defined time period should be divided into fixed and variable categories. Only those costs allocated to the long-term care facility operating department should be included in this analysis. (Refer back to the general discussion of economic considerations for an explanation of cost allocation.)

Inventory holding costs are not included in the break-even analysis for three reasons:
- The stock-in-trade of the pharmacy is, by definition, an income producing asset.
- The value of the inventory carried is a management decision which will affect profitability in a cost analysis.
- Such costs are not expenses of operation separate and above the cost of goods sold and their inclusion as a cost of operation violates generally accepted accounting principles.

A break-even analysis requires estimation of costs and revenues with the variable components of these two figures set at several levels. For example, both costs and revenues vary with the number of prescriptions dispensed. Planning Worksheet #3 provides three columns for listing variable expenses. Column (a) might be used for a low estimate, column (b) for a moderate estimate, and (c) for a high estimate. The variable used could be the number of prescriptions, number of beds, or any measure that is suitable for your situation. In the example in Figure 5-2, the number of prescriptions per year was chosen, so that the average monthly expenses for 1 year could be estimated. Only one column is needed for fixed expenses, because these expenses by definition remain the same regardless of changes in variable expenses. Three columns for total expenses are provided for the three estimates.

Planning Worksheet #4 can be used to compare total revenues with total expenses. It also contains three columns for the low, moderate, and high estimates. The total revenues should be estimated for the same assigned variables chosen for the calculation in Worksheet #3, i.e., number of prescriptions, number of beds, etc. By subtracting the total costs from total revenues, the net profit or loss can be estimated. In the example in Fig. 5-3, the profit and losses calculated reflect estimates for an average month of operation for one year. That is, the profit or loss calculated would be the monthly average for a full year of operation. You may choose any time period that you feel would be useful for your services. It is a prudent idea, however, to monitor actual performance in the first 6 to 12 months very carefully against your estimates. You may wish to project profit and loss for more than three estimates. These estimates are a planning tool to help you predict the economic feasibility of the services you are considering. They will only be as useful as the thought and preparation that you put into them.

A second essential tool in budgeting is a cash flow projection. The object of projecting cash flow is to predict whether sufficient cash will be on hand to pay obligations when they are due. The amount of cash on hand at any time is not the same as the net income estimated in the break-even analysis. Planning Worksheet #5 is a simple form on which you can estimate cash flow. The two sources of cash are your cash reserves or permanent investments and revenue collected. If you are just initiating service, you probably will not collect any revenue for a few weeks or months; therefore the total available cash will come from your cash reserve.

Disbursements are any bills that you must pay. In your initial projection, it would be wise to list cash and disbursements on a daily or weekly basis. By planning cash flow you gain valuable advance notice of cash needs. For example, some of your cash may come from borrowed money. By planning ahead, you can borrow only when needed, and also know when borrowing is indicated. Pharmacists with experience in long-term care say that managing cash flow is one of the greatest challenges, because service to LTCFs is usually provided on a credit basis. Collection of accounts receivable may require 30 days or more. About 60% of long-term care patients are financed by some form of public assistance such as Medicare or Medicaid. Although federal requirements mandate payment of claims within a specified time, the collection process from third-party payers can still be slow and costly. Accordingly, cash flow projections become critical for survival in the marketplace.

## Methods of Cost Recovery

In community pharmacies, revenue is commonly collected by means of a prescription dispensing fee plus ingredient costs for prescription items and by means of a mark-up percentage added on to product costs for other goods. The charge for services provided along with the products is usually included in the dispensing fee. Hospital pharmacies may use a prescription dispensing fee, a per dose for each drug administered, or a per diem charge that includes services and product costs.

Some hospital and community pharmacies provide nondispensing services on a fee for service or hourly rate. The use of a capitation fee in which the pharmacist receives a fixed fee for each patient for a specified period for dispensing and/or nondispensing services exist in both community and hospital pharmacies.

All of these methods of cost recovery are presently used in long-term care pharmacies. In general, you can apply the descriptions, including formulas for calculation, for each method described for hospital and community pharmacies to long-term care practice using the cost estimates arrived at in your planning. Each method has its clerical and management advantages and disadvantages, from the standpoint of calculation, control, adjustment for inflation, or unexpected costs. The American Pharmaceutical Association has supported the use of the professional fee. Some long-term care pharmacists also support the capitation method because in this system revenue is not tied to the drug product. Theoretically, capitation may promote drug product selection and provide an economic incentive, in addition to the legal and professional need, to perform drug utilization and drug regimen review and thereby possibly decrease overall drug utilization.

### Planning Worksheet #3

**BREAK-EVEN ANALYSIS COSTS**

Page _____ of _____

Facility Name _____     Number of Beds _____

| Expense Item (from Column 2 or 3 of Worksheet #2) | Variable Costs (from Columns 5 or 6 of Worksheet #2) | | | Fixed Costs | Total Costs (Variable plus Fixed) | | |
|---|---|---|---|---|---|---|---|
| Defined Variable | a | b | c | | a | b | c |
| 1 | 2 | | | 3 | 4 | | |
| | | | | | | | |
| | | | | | | | |
| | | | | | | | |
| | | | | | | | |
| | | | | | | | |
| | | | | | | | |
| | | | | | | | |
| | | | | | | | |
| | | | | | | | |
| | | | | | | | |
| | | | | | | | |
| | | | | | | | |
| | | | | | | | |
| | | | | | | | |
| | | | | | | | |
| | | | | | | | |
| | | | | | | | |
| | | | | | | | |
| | | | | | | | |
| | | | | | | | |
| | | | | | | | |
| | | | | | | | |
| | | | | | | | |
| | | | | | | | |

Figure 5-2
Sample
## Planning Worksheet #3

### BREAK-EVEN ANALYSIS COSTS

Page ___1___ of ___2___

Facility Name _General YH_                Number of Beds ___100___

| Expense Item (from Column 2 or 3 of Worksheet #2) | Variable Costs (from Columns 5 or 6 of Worksheet #2) | | | Fixed Costs | Total Costs (Variable plus Fixed) | | |
|---|---|---|---|---|---|---|---|
| Defined Variable | a 6480 Rd/yr | b 7200 Rd/yr | c 7920Rd/yr | | a 6480 Rd/yr | b 7200 Rd/yr | c 7920 Rd/yr |
| 1 | | 2 | | 3 | | 4 | |
| Remodeling (written off 12 mos) | | | | ꝑ 117.50 | 117.50 | 117.50 | 117.50 |
| Telephone / month | | | | 12.00 | 12.00 | 12.00 | 12.00 |
| Order forms | 25.92 | 28.80 | 31.68 | | 25.92 | 28.80 | 31.68 |
| Photocopies | 27.00 | 30.00 | 33.00 | | 27.00 | 30.00 | 33.00 |
| Labels | 13.50 | 15.00 | 16.50 | | 13.50 | 15.00 | 16.50 |
| Unit dose mach (3 yrs) | | | | 26.39 | 26.39 | 26.39 | 26.39 |
| Record forms | 7.50 | 8.33 | 9.16 | | 7.50 | 8.33 | 9.16 |
| Pkg supplies | 10.80 | 12.00 | 13.20 | | 10.80 | 12.00 | 13.20 |
| Technician | 287.10 | 319.00 | 351.00 | | 287.10 | 319.00 | 351.00 |
| (Carts (3 yr dep) | | | | 53.33 | 53.33 | 53.33 | 53.33 |
| Misc forms | 2.70 | 3.00 | 3.30 | | 2.70 | 3.00 | 3.30 |
| Book Keeping | 336.60 | 374.00 | 411.40 | | 336.60 | 374.00 | 411.40 |
| Tax @ 5% | 4.37 | 4.86 | 5.35 | | 4.37 | 4.86 | 5.35 |
| General supplies | 18.00 | 20.00 | 22.00 | | 18.00 | 20.00 | 22.00 |
| Pharmacist | | | | 1994.00 | 1994.00 | 1994.00 | 1994.00 |
| Driver | 287.10 | 319.00 | 351.00 | | 287.10 | 319.00 | 351.00 |
| | | | | | | | |
| | | | | | | | |
| Total for page one | 1020.59 | 1133.99 | 1247.59 | 2203.22 | 3223.81 | 3337.21 | 3455.81 |
| | | | | | | | |
| | | | | | | | |
| | | | | | | | |

*The figures in this example are reasonable, but hypothetical. They are used merely to illustrate the planning process.

**Planning Worksheet #4**

BREAK-EVEN ANALYSIS
COST AND REVENUES

Page _____ of _____

Facility Name _____     Number of Beds _____

| Estimates | a | b | c |
|---|---|---|---|
| Revenues | | | |
| | | | |
| | | | |
| | | | |
| | | | |
| Total Revenues | | | |
| Less Total Costs (from Column 4 of Worksheet #3) | | | |
| Net Profit (or Loss) before Taxes | | | |

**Figure 5-3\***
**Sample**
## Planning Worksheet #4
**BREAK-EVEN ANALYSIS**
**COST AND REVENUES**

Page _1_ of _1_

Facility Name _General 7/H_       Number of Beds _100_

| Estimates | a | b | c |
|---|---|---|---|
| _during first year of operation_ | 6450 Rx/yr | 7200 Rx/yr | 7920 Rx/yr |
| **Revenues** | | | |
| _Prescription Revenue_ | 3780.00 | 4200.00 | 4620.00 |
| | | | |
| | | | |
| | | | |
| | | | |
| **Total Revenues** | 3780.00 | 4200.00 | 4620.00 |
| **Less Total Costs** (from Column 4 of Worksheet #3) _from page 2 of estimate_ | 4112.00 | 4225.50 | 4339.10 |
| **Net Profit (or Loss) before Taxes** | (332.10) | (25.50) | 280.90 |

*The figures in this example are reasonable, but hypothetical. They are used merely to illustrate the planning process.

**Planning Worksheet #5**

CASH-FLOW PROJECTION

| | | | | | | | | | | | | |
|---|---|---|---|---|---|---|---|---|---|---|---|---|
| Date | | | | | | | | | | | | |
| Beginning Cash Balance | | | | | | | | | | | | |
| Revenue Collected | | | | | | | | | | | | |
| Total Cash | | | | | | | | | | | | |
| Less Total Disbursements | | | | | | | | | | | | |
| Ending Cash Balance | | | | | | | | | | | | |

In choosing a method of cost recovery, you should weigh all of these factors and choose the most appropriate system for your own situation. If you are providing service for the first time, test a fee system for the first year and change or make adjustments once you have some experience.

## Billing and Collection

Because services to long-term care facilities are provided almost entirely on a credit basis, establishment of effective credit management is essential in your planning activities. Whether patients pay for services from private funds or third parties pay for services, you should be prepared to extend credit and develop and implement a credit collection system. If services are paid by private funds, you may bill patients' responsible agents directly or establish an agreement with the facility to bill patients for you. For patients covered by Medicare, the long-term care facility bills the Medicare agency for all covered services. You are then paid by the facility. In most states, pharmacists are reimbursed directly by the Medicaid program for drugs and related dispensing services. However, the facility bills Medicaid for nondispensing services and reimburses the pharmacist.

The costs associated with offering credit usually consist of soliciting new accounts, investigating credit records, preparing and issuing identification cards, preparing and handling monthly (or more frequent) statements, receiving payments from clients, tracing delinquent accounts, investing capital in accounts receivable, and incurring bad debt expenses. A common problem with credit collection from long-term care facilities and, in particular with third-party programs associated with long-term care, is the length of time required to collect payment. Charges are usually billed monthly but more frequent billing may be desirable. To manage the credit function effectively, you should adhere to a set policy for granting credit and efficiently convert accounts receivable into usable cash.

Proper credit monitoring includes determining the accounts receivable collection period and conducting an aging of accounts analysis. The accounts receivable collection period can be simply calculated by:
- Dividing net credit revenues for a year by the number of days the pharmacy is open to calculate net credit revenues per day
- Dividing the accounts receivable amount from the balance sheet by the net credit revenues per day

The aging of accounts analysis is simply the process of classifying the accounts receivable for a patient by transaction dates. When properly established, this analysis shows the volume of accounts receivable that are current and the volume that are overdue for each patient.

The LTCF may levy service charges for assuming billing, collection, and bad debt losses. The amount of the service charge should be tied to the actual costs and be specified in writing. The costs of collection from patients or governmental agencies probably will not exceed 8% of the monthly charge. The normal and reasonable range is estimated to be between 2.7 and 3.1%.

Ideally, the accounts receivable should be managed very closely to keep the investment in this asset as low as possible and to maximize the cash inflow by using proper billing and collection procedures.

# WHAT COURSE OF ACTION SHOULD I FOLLOW?

Using the plan for service that you have developed, your next step should be to develop a service package that you can present to LTCF administrators. Your service package should include an outline of how your system works, the advantages of it, and samples of forms, reports, equipment, or other features of the system. The administrator is most likely to pay attention to a description of services that are sensitive to his or her perspective—in other words, explain how you are going to help the administrator, not how the LTCF is going to help you. Your description should explain the effect your services will have on the facility, e.g., reduce time nurses spend on drugs, improve and simplify record keeping, reduce errors, reduce waste, and reduce out-of-stock situations.

One possible approach is to develop a standard package of services that is not too detailed. The standard package might contain the basic services that you want to offer, while allowing flexibility to custom design the services for an individual facility. A second alternative would be to develop several clearly defined packages or levels of services and offer the administrator a choice of these packages, retaining the flexibility to mold services to the needs of the facility. A rule-of-thumb to use in presenting choices, however, is to limit them to no more than three options. Offering more than three choices may lead to confusion.

# CONTACTING LTCFS

Your initial contact with administrators might be through provision of a periodic newsletter to interested facilities. Other methods of contact include sending letters and informational material to selected facilities, joining local, state, and national nursing home associations as an associate member, attending meetings, and advertising in local, state, and/or regional nursing home publications. Among the agencies that maintain lists of long-term care facilities are local and state health departments, associations of nursing homes, health care facilties, and homes for the aging, the local office of the Social Security Administration, and the yellow pages of the telephone directory. The initial contact should lead to a personal interview with the administrator and other administrative personnel to present your service packages and evaluate their facility.

Your first meeting with the administrator should leave a favorable impression without being overwhelming or confusing. It may serve to introduce the administrator to your services. You can follow-up with more detail at subsequent meetings. You should not try to force a decision on the administrator. You might wait to be invited back or renew the contact within a few days after the first meeting.

Regardless of the type of service package you offer, your presentation to the administrator should be easy to understand. The administrator should not be confused by what you are offering or overwhelmed by detail, especially at your first meeting. You should leave him or her with confidence of your ability to provide the level of services required, and why you're particularly well suited to provide them. He or she should clearly understand:

- what you propose to do
- how you will do it
- why your package is better
- how much it will cost

Your presentation could be structured sequentially and eventually lead to a no obligation service analysis of the facility. Such an analysis would be beneficial for your planning as well. The forms and analytical procedures suggested previously can be applied to each facility at this point.

If you are successful in reaching an agreement to provide service, the next step is implementation, beginning with preparing a contract. Implementation is covered in Chapter 6.

1. In terms of APhA's *Uniform Cost Accounting System*, each aspect of the pharmacy operation is called an operating department, such as the prescription operating department and nonprescription operating department.

# References for Further Reading

Abraham, A. B., *Analyze Your Records to Reduce Costs*, U.S. Small Business Administration, Washington, D.C., 1978, Publication No. SMA 130.

Barker, P. A., *Budgeting in a Small Service Firm*, U.S. Small Business Administration, Washington, D.C., 1978, Publication No. SMA 146.

Blackwell, R. D., *Knowing Your Image*, U.S. Small Business Administration, Washington, D.C., 1978, Publication No. SMA 124.

Britt, S. H., *Planning Your Advertising Budget*, U.S. Small Business Administration, Washington, D.C., 1978, Publication No. SMA 164.

Campbell, R. K. and J. A. Grisafe, "Study of Prescription Prices and Professional Service," *J. Am. Pharm. Assn., NS17*, 164(1977).

*Checklist for Going into Business*, U.S. Small Business Administration, Washington, D.C., 1978, Publication No. SMA 71.

"Cost of Drugs and Related Medical Supplies," *Medicare Provider Reimbursement Manual*, HIM 15-1, Section 2119, Department of Health, Education, and Welfare, Health Care Financing Administration, July 1978.

Cruger, F. M., *Pointers on Preparing an Employee Handbook*, U.S. Small Business Administration, Washington, D.C., 1978, Publication No. MA 197.

Dickson, W. M. and C. A. Rodowskas, "Research Reporting Allocation of Pharmacist Time for Third Party Prescription Plans," *Inquiry, 12,* 263(1975).

Gagnon, J. P. and C. A. Rodowskas, "Reimbursement Methods for Pharmaceutical Service," *J. Am. Pharm. Assn., NS14*, 675(1974).

Gerson, C. K., "A Growing Trend Toward Fee-for-Service," *Am. Pharm., NS19*, 491(1979).

Halverson, G. B., *Can You Afford Delivery Service?*, U.S. Small Business Administration, Washington, D.C., 1978, Publication No. SMA 133.

Herman, C. and E. Zabloski, "Break-Even Analysis," *Pharm. Manage., 151*, 211(1979).

Kress, G. and R. T. Will, *Marketing Checklist for Small Retailers*, U.S. Small Business Administration, Washington, D.C., 1978, Publication No. SMA 156.

Linckewick, J. A. and F. P. DiMatteo, "A Justification of Unit Dose Drug Distribution from Decentralized Units," *Hosp. Pharm., 13*, 424(1978).

MacStravic, R. E., "Resource Requirements for Health Care Organizations," *Health Care Manage., 4*, 65(Fall 1979).

*Medicare Provider Reimbursement Manual Revision*, Part I, HIM 15-1, Section 2103.1, No. 134, October 1975.

Nelson, A. A., "Calculating the Cost of Filling an Rx," *NARD J., 98*, 20(May 1976).

Nold, E. G. and D. S. Pathak, "Third Party Reimbursement for Clinical Pharmacy Services: Philosophy and Practice," *Am. J. Hosp. Pharm., 34*, 823(1977).

Norwood, G. J. *et al.*, "Reimbursement by Capitation," *Am. Pharm., NS19*, 37(1979).

Oxenfeldt, A. R., "A Decision Making Structure for Price Decisions," *J. Marketing, 37*, 48(1973).

Patterson, L. E. and R. J. Huether, "Reimbursement for Clinical Pharmaceutical Services," *Am. J. Hosp. Pharm., 35*, 1373(1978).

"Reasonable Charges for Prescription Drugs," *Medical Assistance Manual*, Part 6, General Program Administration, 6-160-00, Department of Health, Education, and Welfare, Health Care Financing Administration, p. 36.

Riso, O., *Advertising Guidelines for Small Retail Firms*, U.S. Small Business Administration, Washington, D.C., 1978, Publication No. SMA 160.

Schlissel, M. R., "Pricing in a Service Industry," *M.S.U. Business Topics, 25*, 37(Spring 1977).

Schultz, D. P. *et al.*, "Study Examines Prescription Fees and Services Offered by Pharmacy," *Hospitals, 51*, 78(May 1977).

Siecker, B. R., "Cash Flow Planning and Control in a Pharmacy," *Pharm. Manage., 151*, 260(1979).

Siecker, B. R., *Uniform Cost Accounting System*, Pharmacy Management Institute, American Pharmaceutical Association, Washington, D.C., 1979.

Silverman, M. and M. Lydecker, "Prescription Drug Pricing by Hospital Pharmacies: A Preliminary Study," *Am. J. Hosp. Pharm., 31*, 870(1974).

Smith, H. A., "Determining the Professional Fee," *J. Am. Pharm. Assn., NS8*, 646(1968).

Smith, L. J., *Checklist for Developing a Training Program*, U.S. Small Business Administration, Washington, D.C. 1978, Publication No. SMA 186.

Spaulding, G. *et al.*, "Paying the Pharmacist a Fee for Detecting Adverse Drug Reactions," *J. Am. Pharm. Assn., NS16*, 86(1976).

Strandberg, L. R. *et al.*, "Payment for Nondistributive Hospital Pharmacy Services—a Regional Survey," *Drug Intell. Clin. Pharm., 12*, 410(1978).

Thompson, J. and R. Floyd, "Cost Analysis of Comprehensive Consultant Pharmacist Services in Skilled Nursing Facility: a Progress Report," *Calif. Pharm. (25)*, 22(August 1978).

Tindall, W. N., "Management of Accounts Receivable in the Community Pharmacy," *Till and Tile, 58*, 22(June 1972).

Walker, B. J., *A Pricing Checklist for Small Retailers*, U.S. Small Business Administration, Washington, D.C., 1978, Publication No. SMA 158.

Wantola, Stanley, *Delegating Work and Responsibility*, U.S. Small Business Administration, Washington, D.C., 1978, Publication No. MA 191.

Wertheimer, A. I., "Pricing Pharmaceutical Service—Art, Science or Whim," *J. Am. Pharm. Assn., NS13*, 11(1973).

Wertheimer, A. I., "The Retainer Fee Concept Applied to Pharmacy," *Am. J. Pharm., 144*, 139(1972).

"When the LTCF Assumes Billing and Collecting," *Pharm. Pract., 13*, 84(October 1978).

# Chapter 6:
# IMPLEMENTATION

## WHAT WILL THE CONTRACT CONTAIN?

The first step to implement services in the LTCF is to place all conditions of the service agreement into a written contract.

A written contract defines clearly the duties of each party and provides for administration, evaluation, review, modification, and cancellation. It is written proof of the agreement between two parties. The contract for dispensing service to a LTCF is made between a pharmacy and the LTCF. It should be separate and distinct from the contract between a pharmacist and the LTCF for nondispensing service. In both cases, the contract should be signed by those authorized to enter into such contracts.

Several sources compiled "model" long-term care facility contracts. Often, such models are used improperly. They are completed and filed without due consideration by the facility or the pharmacist. Under such a system, both parties may enter into an agreement that neither really wants. This chapter provides a guideline for you to develop a unique contract.

### Steps in Drafting a Contract

- Each party should obtain the services of an attorney.
- A need for service or desire to provide service is expressed by one party.
- The issues are discussed and compared by both parties.
- A draft contract is prepared and reviewed by the attorneys of both parties.
- If necessary, the draft is modified and then approved by each party.
- The contract is signed and dated by authorized representatives of both parties.
- Copies are distributed to both parties. (A copy of the agreement must be available in the facility for inspection.)
- The contract is reviewed periodically (at least annually).

### Contents of the Contract

#### Contract Between the Facility and the Pharmacy Providing Dispensing Services
1. Identification of Parties

Both the LTCF and the pharmacy providing service should be identified specifically. Qualifications of the pharmacy (such as licensed) should be spelled out. The present size of the facility should be specified to prevent any misunderstanding should it be enlarged. The level of Medicare/Medicaid certification should be listed.

2. Purpose and Objectives of Contract

The contract provides a written record that the pharmacy agrees to provide service to the facility in compliance with all applicable laws and regulations and the policies and procedures of the facility, as may be amended from time to time. In return the facility agrees to certain obligations and considerations.

3. Exchange of Promises and Joint Responsibilities

This is the heart of the agreement and it will probably require a number of separate listings setting forth the functions of both parties. This part of the contract lists the pharmacy's scope of duties. Federal and state regulations establish minimum standards and guidelines. The material contained in earlier chapters contains more information on specific responsibilities. If duties listed are specific fewer problems wil arise during the contract period.

The pharmacy and facility should agree to the facility's medication distribution system and that any major changes in the distribution system should be made by mutual agreement by the two parties.

For example, some of the services the pharmacy may provide are:
- Pharmaceutical service and supplies 24 hours daily, 7 days a week.
- Initial inventory and replenishment of the required drugs in emergency kits.
- Compliance with all state and federal requirements regarding pharmaceutical service in the facility.

The facility should agree to provide the area required for storage of pharmaceuticals and related distribution equipment, preferably at no cost to the provider pharmacy. On-site licensed pharmacy space and rentals should be on a fixed rate agreement and not on a sales percentage or other sliding scale arrangement, to help avoid potential abusive practices. On-site space rent should be commensurate with the prevailing rate for similar space within the community. The contract should specify whether the pharmacy or facility bills private patients.

Unless pharmaceutical service is provided as part of the medical service package offered to patients entering the facility, patients retain the right to freedom of choice of pharmacy.

4. Reasons for Terminating Contract

The agreement should state reasons which justify termination of the contract and how and when the contract may be terminated. Although capricious actions by the facility or pharmacist cannot be completely eliminated, general guidelines should be included to avoid problems.

5. Review, Renewal, and Time Period

The contract should specify the period of time the agreement is to be in effect and also state a requirement that advance notice by either party is necessary before termination or withdrawal from the contract. The date upon which the contract is consumated should be entered. The length of the advance notice required should be dictated in part by the period of time the facility would need to replace the pharmacy if the situation arose. The length of time of the contract is variable, but an annual review and revision would be within reason. Specifying a review of contract terms and retainer amount would be advantageous for dealing with a new administration if one entered while the contract was in force.

6. Insurance

Malpractice insurance is a necessary component for the pharmacist. The amount of insurance coverage should be specific and coordinated with the existing policies of the facility as well as the pharmacy. The party which is to bear the cost of such insurance should be specified and the right, if any, to independent counsel in the event of litigation, should be described.

7. Compensation

The amount and/or the method of calculation of the amount should be specified.

The pharmacy may be reimbursed by private patients on an individual basis. If the facility agrees to act as a billing agent for the pharmacy, the facility may charge for this service. The charges for billing service should be reasonable compared to the prevailing rate for this service in the community.

8. Signatures and Miscellaneous

The written contract should constitute the whole agreement between the facility and the pharmacy. There should be no other agreements, unless signed and appended to the original contract.

The contract should be signed by authorized representatives of both parties and preferably witnessed and/or notarized. If the facility is part of a multiple unit operation some states require separate contracts for each location.

### Contract Between the Facility and the Pharmacist Providing Nondispensing Services

1-3. Refer to the first three sections under the contract for dispensing services. Keep in mind that where the contract for dispensing services referred to the pharmacy, the contract for nondispensing services would refer to the pharmacist.

The services provided by the pharmacist may include pharmaceutical reports, advice, and instructions, as required, in such areas as, but not limited to:

- Committee participation
- Sanitation
- Refrigeration
- Inservice training for facility personnel
- Pharmacy budget
- Drug control, safety, storage, and security
- Patient care policies and monthly medication review
- Compliance with laws and regulations relating to pharmaceutical service

The services provided by the administrator may include, but are not limited to:

- Assurance that the pharmacist has access to all records and supplies necessary for the performance of his or her responsibilities
- Regular meetings with staff and others relative to pharmaceutical procedures

The pharmacist may be temporarily unable to perform these duties, either due to sickness, vacation, or other factors. It is advisable to specify a person capable of immediately serving in the absence of the pharmacist and under what circumstances he or she should be called upon.

4-6. Same as already given.

7. Compensation

The amount and/or the method of calculation of the amount should be specified.

8. Signatures and Miscellaneous

The written contract should constitute the whole agreement between the facility and the pharmacist. There should be no other agreements, unless signed and appended to the original contract.

The contract should be signed by authorized representatives of both parties and preferably witnessed and/or notarized. If the facility is part of a multiple unit operation some states require separate contracts for each location.

# WHAT WILL THE POLICY AND PROCEDURE MANUAL CONTAIN?

While the contract specifies the terms of the agreement and the services to be provided, the policy and procedure manual details the procedures you will follow in providing pharmaceutical service.

A policy and procedure manual is a written guide for personnel, providing specific information on policy decisions and on approved methods and systems for implementing them. It is developed in accordance with the established policies of the facility and serves as an important tool for efficient administration and the upholding of professional standards. In addition, the pharmacy policy and procedure manual can be utilized as a training guide for the facility personnel regarding the scope and intent of pharmacy service provided in the facility. The facility should have policies and procedures covering all of the pharmaceutical service responsibilities listed in Chapters 2–4.

## A Policy Versus a Procedure

A policy is a broad general statement of the course of action (what is to be done) while procedures are how the policy is to be accomplished (approved methods and systems for implementing policies). For example, a policy of storing all medication under approved conditions may have procedures established which specify locked cabinets, controlled temperature, hot and cold running water available at or near the storage area, and separate storage for external medications.

The policy and procedures combined should answer the following questions about every activity:

| | |
|---|---|
| What is its purpose? | RE: Policy statement |
| Why is it necessary? | RE: Policy statement |
| Where should it be done? | RE: Nursing stations, medication, storage room, etc. |
| When should it be done? | RE: Time limits, time of day, etc. |
| Who should do it? | RE: M.D., R.N., Nurses Aide, R.Ph. |
| How should it be done? | RE: Specificity of statement |

## Developing a Policy and Procedure Manual

Since procedures are a process and implementation of policies, it need not be important to separate the two statements. Many procedures are in effect describing the policy as well, yet each policy has a procedure. Obviously, the more specific a policy becomes, the more of a procedure it becomes. Often the policy will be the key sentence to the procedure.

Experience shows that committing to writing those existing and approved procedures is, perhaps, the easiest approach to a formalized policy and procedure manual.

• Who should write the procedure?

Generally, the person who performs the procedure writes the most clear and accurate activity description. Each manual should be individually developed and constructed to reflect the policies and procedures of a particular facility.

• Seek simplicity.

Elimination of unnecessary details and combination of similar elements will result in a readable, easy-to-interpret manual.

• Decide on a format and keep it simple.

Numbering all pages sequentially may be troublesome for updating purposes. You may use a numbering sequence of "1.0, 1.1, 1.2, 1.3, etc. . . ." "2.0, 2.1, 2.2, 2.3, etc. . . ." for each subtopic covered. This facilitates easy reference and revision.

• Develop a sequence of presenting procedures.

The presentation of the procedure in the way it is actually performed is the most logical method to follow. The Table of Contents of the manual provides the guideline of policy and procedure sequence. Each procedure should be presented in a similar manner, whether it be in an outline, flow chart, or narrative form.

• Envision a method for changes and revisions from the beginning.

Regulations require periodic updating of the manual. A format which makes updating simple is a three-ring, loose leaf binder with indexed dividers between the separate topics. Each individual topic will comprise a chapter, the pages of which are numbered with the sequence described above. The Table of Contents should include a section describing the time-table for periodic revisions and updates.

• Include actual forms.

Inclusion of those forms actually used in-house complements the procedures but does not replace the narrative. The forms should be completed to represent an actual procedure in action. For example, the physician's order form, properly submitted to the pharmacy, may be accompanied by the completed nurse's cardex, the medication cards, and the form used to transmit information to the pharmacist.

The list of procedures described in Chapters 2–4 may be used as a guide for developing the policy and procedure manual. The procedures used to implement policies are determined by the system of drug distribution utilized and other operating procedures in the facility. They must be tailored specifically for each facility.

# How To Use a Policy and Procedure Manual

The specific purpose of the manual is to provide uniform standards for quality pharmaceutical care to patients served by the LTC facility. The manual facilitates improved patient care by enabling the administrator to have a better understanding of the requirements for providing high standards of pharmaceutical service and a greater appreciation of the level of care provided by the pharmacist and the pharmacy.

- To the nursing staff the manual offers a clear and systematic procedure for performing drug-related patient care services.
- To the physician who wishes a prescribed drug therapy program to be carried out properly, the manual provides those standards to ensure this outcome.
- To the pharmacist, the manual will serve as a guideline for providing quality pharmaceutical service to patients in the facility.

Implementation of the standards described in the manual should result in an effective drug use control system in the facility. A well-used manual with "dog-eared" pages indicates that the staff is making day-to-day reference to provide consistently high quality health care services to the residents of the home.

The Policy and Procedure Manual should accomplish the following.

**Promotion of consistent service.**

For accessibility and clarity of procedures, the manual affords excellent assistance to the nursing staff which may at times have difficulty reaching the physician or pharmacist.

**Promotion of team work.**

By outlining the required activities of each segment of the facility staff, e.g., R.N., nurse's aide, pharmacist, the team approach is encouraged. If the level of expectation is spelled out, a smooth performance of duties may be seen by the members of the health care team.

**Provision of excellent information for training new employees and continuing education of other employees.**

Inservice training sessions, held for only new employees or with present staff, are recommended. It is important for all those who are expected to carry out the policies and procedures to know what their respective duties are. If the training sessions are held regularly for orientation of new employees only, this should be so stated in the manual. Using the manual for this purpose ensures continuity of training as changes in staff occur.

**Establishment of standards against which actual performance can be measured.**

Several additional non-patient related applications of the manual are evident: (a) the personnel department may wish to identify those staff members not meeting standards of performance, and (b) in litigation cases concerning substandard performance, the manual contains those guidelines against which the questionable performance can be measured.

**Provision of a means for comparing competent practice to written approved procedures.**

If current practices do not follow the procedures in the manual, perhaps a review and revision is in order. The standards should reflect the actual operating procedures in the facility.

**Provision of a central source for adding, deleting, or changing policy or procedures.**

The manual available to all personnel provides an excellent method of improving staff awareness and decreases the confusion which could affect the services provided the residents.

**Improvement of inter- and intradepartmental communications and working relationships.**

Misunderstandings among a facility's staff can lead to ill-feelings and a poor working relationship. Concisely stated policies and procedures can prevent misdirected blame and confusion among the members of the health care team.

**Prevention of errors resulting from the verbal transmission of policy and procedures from one employee to another.**

Proper documentation of directions is a necessity for good patient care. In the busy routine of everyday pharmacy and nursing practice, verbal orders can be easily misinterpreted. The policy and procedures manual can serve as a standard guide and reference to the facility's staff.

## Approval Required

Preceding the use of a formalized set of policies and procedures encompassed in the manual, approval of the administrative body of the facility should be sought. The medical staff should have input through the Pharmaceutical Service Committee, which has the overall responsibility for the development of the manual. Also considered should be adequate means for evaluation and compliance. As previously stated, the updating timetable is best incorporated in the Table of Contents. The manual should be updated at least annually.

## Quality Assurance Aid

The manual provides a quality assurance tool for pharmaceutical service. It outlines areas of current accountability and gives a yardstick of quality of service. The pharmacist may wish to review his or her own services and point out gaps in continuity for which manual revisions are necessary. Evaluation of current practices may suggest methods for improvement.

## Promotes Efficiency

Efficient use of personnel is one of the strong points of a policy and procedure manual. Delegation of authority not only outlines areas of control but frees supervisory personnel from repetitive explanations of procedures. It is imperative that the document be distributed within the facility where the most beneficial use can be achieved; e.g., nursing stations, physician care area, and administrative offices.

## Standards Set

Standards of practice are established in the manual which may be reviewed in depth by licensing, regulating, and accreditating agencies. From their point of view, the manual ensures compliance with the various standards, and performance within the facility is measurable against these standards. If pharmacy practice standards state that "24-hour service is provided," it is important to ensure that this service is provided. *Do what you say you do* is an important point to remember when developing a policy and procedure manual.

## Distribution and Interpretation

Proper distribution and interpretation of the manual for all employees is stressed. A distribution list should be kept to update *all* copies available. It is best to clarify where the manual is available in the front of the manual, with specific locations identified. For example, the locations cited should include: all patient care areas, nursing stations, physicians' offices, dispensing areas (if an on-premise pharmacy is established), central nursing office, medication rooms, and, of course, in the pharmacist's possession.

## Role Clarification

The pharmacist's role should be spelled out in both the nursing and medical policy and procedure manuals. This leads to greater acceptance of the team concept of health care and clarifies areas of overlapping procedures.

## Summary

In summary, the policy and procedure manual provides an approach for various health care providers to work together in a concerted effort and a common goal—to improve the care of their patients.

# HOW WILL I CONTROL AND EVALUATE SERVICES?

Periodic review and assessment, followed by modification of service or corrective action when necessary, should be an integral part of service to each facility. The scope of review may encompass assurance of compliance with laws, regulations, and good practice standards as well as an assessment of the efficiency of service. The skilled nursing facility regulations require that the pharmacist provide a written report at least quarterly to the pharmaceutical services committee on the status of the facility's pharmaceutical services and staff performance, and it is recommended that this standard be applied to other levels of care as well, to be used in the assessment process.

Changes may occur in the laws and regulations. Changes may occur in the size and staffing of the facility. Any of these changes would affect the climate in which service is provided and require modification of the services or procedures.

To make adjustments to account for such changes, you should:

- Be alert to changes that come about in pharmaceutical service, long-term care, and in the facility,
- Check procedures against these changes,
- Determine the revisions, if any that are needed.

Control and evaluation require several types of documentation. One form of documentation are the records routinely maintained in the facility and pharmacy, such as patient medication profiles, medication administration records, and drug use control sheets. Documentation should also include a record of the time spent providing service and periodic review of the total status of service.

## Documentation of Time

In providing service, you make a commitment to devote sufficient time to establish quality service to the facility. Just as an employer maintains a record of the time spent by workers, the LTCF may desire a record of the time spent by you and the supportive personnel to document that adequate time is being spent to fulfill the agreement for service to the facility. The information in this record may also be used as the basis for you to determine staffing needs for performing service and the appropriate amount of compensation for service.

Throughout this book pharmaceutical service is divided into dispensing and nondispensing services. These services are further subdivided into various functions which pharmacists may perform in serving long-term care patients. The time spent in performing dispensing functions should be recorded separately from time for nondispensing functions. In all cases, the facility should have an agreement with a pharmacy for dispensing service and a separate agreement with a pharmacist for nondispensing service such that separate documentation would be required.

At times you may desire a record of activity which breaks the functions down into more specific categories. A detailed categorization of activity is useful when initially establishing service and to reassess periodically how time is spent to assure that activities are organized efficiently.

The categorization of service suggested in this section is flexible. The broad categories may be used for routine recording of time required for pharmaceutical service to the facility. The more specific categories may be used for more detailed time studies. Since no one activity can be performed exclusive of all others, there is always the problem of overlapping actions in any categorization. Nevertheless, the breakdown should assist you in recording, with greater accuracy, information in a format which will give a more useful picture of how

Figure 6-1

# Pharmaceutical Service Activities Record Code

1.0 Dispensing Services

1.1 Receipt of Drug Order
1. Recording and Interpretation of Order
2. Consultation with Physician or Nurse Concerning Order
3. Enforcement of Stop Order Policy

1.2 Maintenance of Patient Medication Profile

1.3 Labeling and Dispensing the Drug Order

1.4 Delivery of Drugs

1.5 Storage of Drugs
1. Maintenance of Storage Area in Facility
2. Emergency Kit Maintenance

1.6 Accountability of Drugs
1. Maintenance of Control Records
2. Disposition of Drugs

2.0 Nondispensing Services

2.1 Administration of Drugs

2.2 Review of Drug Regimen
1. Monthly Audit
2. Preparation of Reports

2.3 Participation on Committees
1. Pharmaceutical Services
2. Utilization Review
3. Infection Control
4. Patient Care Policy

2.4 Inservice Education
1. Preparing and Presenting Programs
2. Preparation of Newsletter
3. Attending Other Programs

2.5 Patient Discharge Counselling

3.0 Miscellaneous

3.1 Participation in Continuing Education

3.2 Billing and Collection

**Figure 6-2**

## PHARMACEUTICAL SERVICE ACTIVITIES RECORD

Period from _7/7_ to ___ 19 ___.
Record of: _Al Smith_     For: _Southside PH_

| Activity (code) | Time (minutes) | Date 7/7 | | | | | | | | | | | | | | | Total |
|---|---|---|---|---|---|---|---|---|---|---|---|---|---|---|---|---|---|
| 1.11 | | 80 | | | | | | | | | | | | | | | 80 |
| 1.12 | | 5 | | | | | | | | | | | | | | | 5 |
| 1.3 | | 10 | | | | | | | | | | | | | | | 10 |
| 1.2 | | 80 | | | | | | | | | | | | | | | 80 |
| 2.2 | | 60 | | | | | | | | | | | | | | | 60 |
| 2.5 | | 15 | | | | | | | | | | | | | | | 15 |
| 2.31 | | 60 | | | | | | | | | | | | | | | 60 |
| | | | | | | | | | | | | | | | TOTAL | | 200 |

### TOTAL NUMBER OF MINUTES BY CATEGORY

| 1.00 | 2.00 | 3.00 | Total | | | | |
|---|---|---|---|---|---|---|---|
| 65 | 135 | | 200 | | | | |

## PHARMACEUTICAL SERVICE ACTIVITIES RECORD

Period from _7/7_ to ___ 19 ___.
Record of: _Sue Jones_     For: _Southside PH_

| Activity (code) | Time (minutes) | Date 7/7 | | | | | | | | | | | | | | | Total |
|---|---|---|---|---|---|---|---|---|---|---|---|---|---|---|---|---|---|
| 1.3 | | 120 | | | | | | | | | | | | | | | 120 |
| | | | | | | | | | | | | | | | | | |
| | | | | | | | | | | | | | | | | | |
| | | | | | | | | | | | | | | | | | |
| | | | | | | | | | | | | | | | | | |
| | | | | | | | | | | | | | | | | | |
| | | | | | | | | | | | | | | | TOTAL | | 120 |

### TOTAL NUMBER OF MINUTES BY CATEGORY

| 1.00 | 2.00 | 3.00 | Total | | | | |
|---|---|---|---|---|---|---|---|
| 120 | | | 120 | | | | |

Developed by: American Pharmaceutical Association

your time is spent from which the data can be readily retrieved for analysis. The same code may be used for documenting your activity and the supportive personnel.

The activities code in Fig. 6-1 may be used with various record forms. Two examples of use of time documentation follow, in Fig. 6-2 and 6.3.

## Example Situation

Alan Smith is a pharmacist at the Medical Center Pharmacy. He serves two nursing homes. This morning, July 7, the medication orders from Southside Nursing Home are received for dispensing.

Mr. Smith first checks the orders for accuracy and completeness (20 minutes, Code 1.11). He has a question concerning the strength of one medication, so he contacts the nurse at the facility (5 minutes, Code 1.12). Sue Jones, Mr. Smith's assistant, spends 2 hours dispensing and labeling the medication orders (120 minutes, Code 1.3). Mr. Smith checks the completed orders (10 minutes, Code 1.3) and updates the in-pharmacy medication records (30 minutes, Code 1.2).

Later that day, Mr. Smith is at the facility. He spends 1 hour reviewing a selected number of charts (60 minutes, Code 2.2) and reviews the instructions for taking medications with a patient who is to be discharged later that day (15 minutes, Code 2.5).

In the evening, Mr. Smith attends a meeting of the Pharmaceutical Service Committee of Southside Nursing Home. He has prepared and presents a plan for improving handling of controlled substances in the facility (60 minutes, Code 2.31).

If Mr. Smith desires to make an in-depth study of the use of time in providing service to the facility, he might utilize the first form illustrated (Figure 6-2) to record his activities and those of his assistant. For a less detailed, daily record of activity, he could use the second form illustrated (Figure 6-3). These forms may be retained in a loose-leaf notebook.

Some pharmacists find that a bound notebook kept as a log book is more practical than retention of records on loose-leaf paper.

A summary of pharmacists' activities may be made monthly and recorded on a form.

## Pharmaceutical Services Checklist

The Pharmaceutical Service Checklist describes components of pharmaceutical service which should be inspected in each periodic review of the actual status of service. The Checklist does not suggest the criteria for rating each item. You should develop a set of criteria based on experience and information provided in the facility's policies and procedures manual. A few items may be assessed easily. For example, whether proper temperature is maintained in the medication room or drug cabinet may be checked by a look at the thermometer kept in the drug room. Other items may not be as easy to evaluate. For example, to determine whether stop order procedures are adequate, you would need to examine other elements of patient care, such as appropriateness of drug therapy through drug regimen review. To determine if stop order procedures are being followed, you may look at drug order and administration records.

You should perform a quarterly quality control review of the facility's pharmaceutical services. The review should include, but not be limited to, an inspection of each nursing station, its related drug storage area, patient's health records, and staff performance. The checklist report may be used as a portion of the review documentation. A copy should be posted in the corresponding medicine room. A copy should be provided for the administrator, director of nursing service, and pharmacist.

A summary monthly report may be prepared from the quality control review and the monthly drug regimen reviews. In some facilities, an exit conference with the pharmacist, administrator, and director of nursing services is held within a reasonable period after the quarterly review is performed. The quality control summary report indicating findings and recommendations is submitted by the pharmacist at the exit conference. An appropriate target date of correction and plan of implementation are established for each finding.

Where possible, an inservice training session by the pharmacist is scheduled with the facility staff after the exit conference to review the quality control report and plan of correction.

A copy of the quality control summary report is usually submitted to the pharmaceutical services committee, administrator, and the director of nursing services. This report is forwarded at least quarterly. Figure 6-4 is an example of a quality control summary report form. Figure 6-5 is the Pharmaceutical Service Checklist.

Figure 6-3

### Pharmaceutical Service Activities Record

Period From: _7/7_ to _____ 19 _____ .
Record of: _Lil Smith_ For: _Northside NH_

**Total Number of Hours by Category**

| Date | 1.00 | 2.00 | 3.00 | Total |
|------|------|------|------|-------|
| 7/7 | 65/60 | 135/60 | | 200/60 |
| | | | | |
| Total | 65/60 | 135/60 | | 200/60 |

### Pharmaceutical Service Activities Record

Period From: _7/7_ to _____ 19 _____ .
Record of: _Sue Jones_ For: _Northside NH_

**Total Number of Hours by Category**

| Date | 1.00 | 2.00 | 3.00 | Total |
|------|------|------|------|-------|
| 7/7 | 120/60 | | | 120/60 |
| | | | | |
| Total | 120/60 | | | 120/60 |

**Figure 6-4**

## PHARMACIST COORDINATOR
### QUALITY CONTROL SUMMARY REPORT

*DATE:* _____

*Facility №* _____

*Coordinator* _____

| REFERENCE | DATE | FINDINGS | RECOMMENDATIONS | TARGET DATE CORRECTION | FOLLOW-UP |
|-----------|------|----------|-----------------|------------------------|-----------|
|  |  |  |  |  |  |
|  |  |  |  |  |  |
|  |  |  |  |  |  |
|  |  |  |  |  |  |
|  |  |  |  |  |  |
|  |  |  |  |  |  |
|  |  |  |  |  |  |
|  |  |  |  |  |  |
|  |  |  |  |  |  |
|  |  |  |  |  |  |
|  |  |  |  |  |  |
|  |  |  |  |  |  |
|  |  |  |  |  |  |

Figure 6-5

## Pharmaceutical Services Checklist

|  | Yes | No | Comments |
|---|---|---|---|

**General**

1. The policy and procedures manual is current.
2. The pharmacist's service agreement is current.
3. The pharmacy's service agreement is current.
4. Administrator, nurses and/or other facility personnel are interviewed for existing or potential problems.

**Dispensing Services**

1. Receipt of Medication Order

   a Records are properly kept for ordered medications from the pharmacy.

   b Renewals of prescriptions, especially for maintenance medications, are ordered appropriately without interruption of therapy.

   c Direct copies of physician orders are forwarded to the pharmacy.

   d Written copies of all telephone medication orders are promptly sent to the prescribing physician for signature.

   e The signed copies of telephone orders are included in the patient's chart.

   f Medication orders are recapped or rewritten monthly, when appropriate, and signed by the physician.

   g Medication orders are properly written.

   h Medication orders in the patient's chart concur with those on the medication administration sheet.

   i Specific nurses are authorized to transmit medication orders from the patient's chart to the pharmacy.

   j A list of approved abbreviations is posted and used in medication orders.

   k Each physician on staff has been informed of the stop order policy.

   l A copy of the stop order policy is posted in the medicine room.

   m The stop order procedures are adequate and being followed.

2. Maintenance of Patient Profile

   a The pharmacy maintains an individual medication record for all drugs dispensed for each patient, including quantities, renewals, etc.

   b The patient profile includes a medication history of prescription and nonprescription drugs taken from the patient's medical records or by patient interview.

3. Labeling and Dispensing the Medication Order

   a The compounding, packaging, and dispensing of drugs is performed by a pharmacist or under his or her supervision.

   b Medication labels are clearly and properly prepared.

   c Medication labels are not altered or re-used.

   d Non-legend drugs are properly labeled.

   e Date of reconstitution is listed on vials or containers.

|  |  | Yes | No | Comments |
|---|---|---|---|---|
| f | The procedure for updating medication labels is being followed. | ___ | ___ | _____ |
| g | Multidose vials of injectable drugs are dated when first used. | ___ | ___ | _____ |

4. Delivery of Medication Order

| a | A schedule of pharmacy operating hours and ordering times is posted at the nursing station. | ___ | ___ | _____ |
|---|---|---|---|---|
| b | The delivery schedule is adequate and is being met. | ___ | ___ | _____ |
| c | The 24-hour emergency telephone number of each pharmacy is posted at the nursing station. | ___ | ___ | _____ |
| d | The emergency service meets the needs of the patients. | ___ | ___ | _____ |

5. Storage of Medications

| a | The utility room or cabinet containing poisons and cleaning supplies is locked. | ___ | ___ | _____ |
|---|---|---|---|---|
| b | Medications are stored in a locked cabinet or room that is not accessible to patients or visitors. | ___ | ___ | _____ |
| c | The keys to the medicine room or drug cabinet are under the control of the nurse. | ___ | ___ | _____ |
| d | Unauthorized personnel are not permitted to enter or use the drug storage area. | ___ | ___ | _____ |
| e | The proper temperature (15-30 °C) is maintained in the medication room or drug cabinet. | ___ | ___ | _____ |
| f | Drug administration areas are well lighted. | ___ | ___ | _____ |
| g | Medication counters in the drug room or drug cabinets are clean and uncluttered. | ___ | ___ | _____ |
| h | A metric-apothecary conversion chart is posted in the medication storage area. | ___ | ___ | _____ |
| i | Discontinued and outdated drugs are properly marked, stored and appropriately disposed of. | ___ | ___ | _____ |
| j | Non-drug items are not stored in the drug storage area. | ___ | ___ | _____ |
| k | Medications are stored in the original containers. There is no transfer of medications between containers. | ___ | ___ | _____ |
| l | Special containers are used for appropriate medications to prevent deterioration. | ___ | ___ | _____ |
| m | There is no evidence of excessive quantities of drugs. | ___ | ___ | _____ |
| n | The nursing station has adequate supplies for the proper storage and administration of medications. | ___ | ___ | _____ |
| o | There are no drugs requiring refrigeration in the cubicles. | ___ | ___ | _____ |
| p | The proper temperature (2-15 °C) for refrigerated items is being maintained. | ___ | ___ | _____ |
| q | Drugs requiring low temperatures are the only medications kept in the refrigerator. | ___ | ___ | _____ |
| r | Outdated drugs are removed from the refrigerator. | ___ | ___ | _____ |
| s | Only adjuncts to medication administration are stored in the refrigerator with medications. | ___ | ___ | _____ |
| t | Medications for external use only are stored separately away from medications for internal use. | ___ | ___ | _____ |

|  | Yes | No | Comments |
|---|---|---|---|

5.1   Controlled Substances

     a   Controlled drugs are not accessible to nonauthorized personnel.     ____ ____ _____

     b   Schedule II controlled drugs are stored in a locked cabinet or drawer separate from non-Schedule II drugs.     ____ ____ _____

5.2   Emergency Kit

     a   The emergency medication kit is stored in an area known to personnel handling medications, and is readily accessible.     ____ ____ _____

     b   A list of the contents of the emergency kit is posted near the telephone at the nursing station.     ____ ____ _____

     c   The emergency medication kit is properly sealed.     ____ ____ _____

     d   The drugs in the emergency kit have not expired.     ____ ____ _____

     e   The use of the emergency kit is properly recorded in a log book.     ____ ____ _____

     f   A letter regarding use of the emergency drug supply has been sent to each staff physician.     ____ ____ _____

     g   The emergency kit contents have been checked monthly by the pharmacist.     ____ ____ _____

5.3   Bedside Medications

     a   The bedside storage of medications is specifically ordered by the patient's physician.     ____ ____ _____

     b   Medications are properly labeled for bedside use.     ____ ____ _____

     c   The patient has been properly instructed on the use of bedside medication.     ____ ____ _____

6.   Accountability of Medications

     a   A formulary has been developed and approved for those items to be considered as house (or stock) supply items. PRN OTC's are the only approved stock items where no in-house pharmacy exists.     ____ ____ _____

     b   Control procedures have been established and are followed for drugs brought in by newly admitted patients, physician samples, and investigational drugs.     ____ ____ _____

     c   All medications sent with the patient on discharge have been properly ordered by the physician and recorded in the patient's records.     ____ ____ _____

     d   All discharge medications are properly labeled and packaged.     ____ ____ _____

6.1   Schedule II Controlled Substances

     a   Separate records are maintained for Schedule II controlled drugs.     ____ ____ _____

     b   Schedule II controlled drugs are destroyed in the presence of a registered pharmacist and a registered nurse employed by the facility according to federal and state regulations.     ____ ____ _____

     c   Proper records are kept for controlled drugs destroyed in the facility.     ____ ____ _____

6.2   Disposition of Medication

     a   Drug disposal is properly documented.     ____ ____ _____

     b   Drugs not used or re-ordered within 90 days are removed from the cubical and disposed of.     ____ ____ _____

| **Nondispensing Services** | Yes | No | Comments |
|---|---|---|---|

1. Administration of Medications

   a Administration of routine medications is properly recorded in each patient's record.  _____  _____  _____

   b Administration of PRN medications is properly recorded in each patient's health record.  _____  _____  _____

   c There is not a significant number of PRN medications being administered on a regular basis, for more than two weeks.  _____  _____  _____

   d All medications are prepared, administered and charted by the same licensed person.  _____  _____  _____

   e Only licensed or authorized personnel administer medications.  _____  _____  _____

   f There is no evidence of borrowing medications from one patient and administering to another.  _____  _____  _____

   g When drugs are removed from the original containers, they are maintained in environments ensuring proper purity and potency up to the time of administration.  _____  _____  _____

   h The procedures and equipment used in drug administration provide for accurate drug dosage, identification, and sanitation.  _____  _____  _____

   i There is no evidence of pre-charting doses before administration.  _____  _____  _____

   j The time interval between prescribed doses and actual administration falls within a range of two hours.  _____  _____  _____

   k The procedure for monitoring and recording medication errors has been implemented and adhered to.  _____  _____  _____

2. Review of Drug Regimen

   a The pharmacist has submitted a written quarterly report for the last quarter.  _____  _____  _____

   b The pharmacist reviews each patient's drug regimen every thirty days.  _____  _____  _____

   c The pharmacist provides documentation of the results (follow-up) of irregularity reports.  _____  _____  _____

   d The pharmacist maintains a record of all visits and activities in the facility.  _____  _____  _____

3. Participation on Committees

   a The Committee on Pharmaceutical Service has met this quarter.  _____  _____  _____

   b The Utilization Review Committee has met this quarter.  _____  _____  _____

   c The Infection Control Committee has met this quarter.  _____  _____  _____

   d The Patient Care Policy Committee has met this quarter.  _____  _____  _____

4. Provision of Inservice Training

   a The pharmacist provides an inservice training program on a regularly scheduled basis.  _____  _____  _____

   b Documentation of inservice training is available.  _____  _____  _____

5. Patient Discharge Counseling

   a The pharmacist provides instruction to discharged patients concerning their medication therapy when appropriate.  _____  _____  _____

# References for Further Reading

Archambault, G.F., "Documentation Used by Surveyors to Evaluate Pharmacies Servicing Non-hospitalized Patients," *J. Clin. Pharm., 2,* 532(1977).

Farmer, R.A. and Associates, *What You Should Know About Contracts,* Arco Publishing Co., Inc., 219 Park Avenue South, New York, NY 10003, 1969.

Fink, J.L. III, "Liability of Pharmacists Serving Skilled Nursing Facilities," *J. Am. Pharm. Assn., NS17,* 95(1977).

Jones, E.W. *et al., Assesing the Quality of Long-Term Care,* National Center for Health Services Research, Research Summary Series, U.S. Department of Health, Education, and Welfare, Public Health Service, Pub. No. (PHS) 78-3192, 1978.

Linn, M.W. *et al.,* "Patient Outcome as a Measure of Quality Nursing Home Care," *Am. J. Public Health, 67,* 337(1977).

Lowe, M.A. and J.A. Lowe, "If It Isn't Documented It Isn't Done," *Am. Health Care Assn. J., 5,* 71(1979).

Reader's Digest, *You and the Law,* The Reader's Digest Association, Inc., Pleasantville, New York, 1973, pp. 196-217.

Ross, M.J., *Handbook of Everyday Law,* 3rd ed., Harper and Row Publishers, New York, NY 10022, 1975, pp. 20-63.

Zimmer, J.G., "Medical Care Evaluation Studies in Long-Term Care Facility," *J. Am. Ger. Soc., 27,* 62-72 (February 1979).

# Appendix

## I. How to Obtain Copies of Standards

### Federal Regulations for Long-Term Care Facilities

The federal Medicare and Medicaid regulations for Skilled Nursing and Intermediate Care Facilities are listed in the *Code of Federal Regulations* under the following titles and sections:

Title 42 Public Health, Part IV Health Care Financing Administration, Department of Health and Human Services (Parts 400-499).

The Conditions of Participation for Skilled Nursing Facilities are listed in sections 405.1101 to 405.1137. The Standards for Intermediate Care Facilities other than facilities for the mentally retarded are listed in sections 442.300 to 442.346. The Standards for Intermediate Care Facilities for the Mentally Retarded are listed in sections 442.400 to 442.516.

Title 42 is updated each year and a new volume is issued approximately every October. For inquiries concerning the most recent edition, its availability, and price, write to Director, Office of Federal Register, National Archives and Records Service, General Services Administration, Washington, D.C. 20408 or call (202) 523-5240. Copes of the *Code* are sold by the Superintendent of Documents, Government Printing Office, Washington, DC 20402.

### Joint Commission on the Accreditation of Hospitals (JCAH)

The JCAH has published an *Accreditation Manual for Long Term Care Facilties.* For information on the most recent edition of the Manual available, write to the JCAH, 875 North Michigan Avenue, Chicago, IL 60611.

### Other Regulations and Standards for Long-Term Care Facilities

State and local laws and regulations should be obtained from the appropriate state or local agency, usually called the state department of health or local health department. Information on standards published by private organizations should be obtained from the responsible organization. A list of several national long-term care organizations follows.

American Association of Homes for the Aging
1050 17th Street, N.W.
Washington, DC 20036

American College of Nursing Home Administrators
4650 East West Highway
Washington, DC 20014

American Health Care Association
1200 15th Street, NW
Washington, DC 20005

National Council of Health Care Services
2600 Virginia Ave., NW, Suite 915
Washington, DC 20037

### Long-Term Care Statistics

The National Center for Health Statistics conducts periodic surveys of the nation's long-term care facilities. The results of these surveys are published in Series 13—Data on Health Resources Utilization and Series 14—Data on Health Resources: Manpower and Facilities. Information on available publications can be obtained by writing to: Scientific and Technical Information Branch, National Center for Health Statistics, Public Health Service, Hyattsville, MD 20782.

## II. APhA and American Health Care Association Approved Joint Statement on Pharmaceutical Service in the Long-Term Care Facility

(The Board of Trustees of the American Pharmaceutical Association and the Board of Directors of the American Health Care Association (formerly the American Nursing Home Association) have both formally approved a joint Statement on Pharmaceutical Service in the Long-Term Care Facility (August 1976). The statement was drafted by the Liaison Committee which has existed between the two associations for a number of years. The statement is designed to clarify the relationships which should exist between a pharmacist and a facility particularly as it relates to compensation for service. The statement follows.)

It is the responsibility of the long-term care facility to ensure that pharmaceutical service is provided in accordance with accepted professional principles and appropriate federal, state, and local laws and regulations. Pharmaceutical service is under the general supervision of a qualified pharmacist who is responsible to the administrator for developing, coordinating and supervising all aspects of pharmaceutical services within the long-term care facility. The pharmacist serving in this capacity may or may not dispense drug products to patients in the facility.

If the pharmacist is not a salaried employee of the facility, the responsibilities of both parties must be properly delineated in a written agreement between the pharmacist and the facility. In the agreement for the provision of pharmaceutical services, it is essential that all considerations between the pharmacist and the long-term care facility be carefully and precisely specified.

The pharmacist, by reason of professional and legal criteria, has certain responsibilities to all persons to whom drug products are dispensed, whether the recipient of the drug product resides within or outside of a long-term care facility. The pharmacist has additional responsibilities relating to those who reside in the long-term care facility as a result of regulations promulgated by federal and state agencies. Compensation to the pharmacist for the fulfillment of the responsibilities outlined in the agreement shall be determined by negotiation between the pharmacist and the facility representative.

Charges for drug products and dispensing services may be made directly by the pharmacist to the party who has fiscal responsibility for the recipient, or such charges may be forwarded to the long-term care facility for collection and remittance to the pharmacist. In those instances where the facility provides the billing and collection services, the facility should bill the pharmacist on a separate invoice for a mutually acceptable and reasonable accounting and collection fee which covers cost experienced by the facility for assuming bill collection including bad debt and other normal accounting responsibility.

## III.  Joint Commission on Accreditation of Hospitals Standards for Pharmaceutical Services in Long-Term Care Facilities (reprinted with permission from *Accreditation Manual for Long-Term Care Facilities*, 1980, Chicago, Ill.)

### Principle

The facility shall assure the availability of pharmaceutical services that are conducted in accordance with accepted ethical and professional practices and that meet all applicable federal, state, and local laws and rules and regulations.

### Standard I

The facility shall be responsbile for obtaining all drugs and biologicals required by patients/residents in the facility. The scope of pharmaceutical services, including available drugs and biologicals, shall be commensurate with the medication needs of the patients/residents.

The facility shall make drugs and biologicals available by one of the following methods.
- A licensed pharmacy within the facility,
- Agreement with an outside licensed pharmacy(ies), or
- A combination of the above.

The facility shall provide an emergency medication kit.

### Standard II

All pharmaceutical services within the facility shall be under the general supervision of a licensed pharmacist who is responsible to the administration for developing, coordinating, and monitoring all pharmaceutical services.

If the facility does not employ a pharmacist on a full-time or part-time basis, the facility shall have a written agreement with a consultant pharmacist to monitor the pharmaceutical services within the facility.

The pharmacist shall be currently licensed to practice pharmacy by the state in which he or she is practicing and should have formal training or one year of experience in the specialized functions performed by pharmaceutical services in a long-term care facility.

The pharmacist shall be responsible for the control of all drugs and biologicals used in the facility. Controls shall be established that assure compliance with federal, state, and local laws and rules and regulations.

The pharmacist must assure that drug records are in order and that an account of all controlled drugs is maintained. The pharmacist shall also ensure that all drugs are properly labeled and stored.

The pharmacist shall perform a monthly review of each patient's/resident's drug regimen for any potential interactions, interferences, or incompatibilities, and for other pertinent information. The pharmacist shall indicate in the patient's/resident's medical record that he or she has performed the review and sign and date the entry. Any irregularities shall be reported in writing to the attending physician, the medical director, and the administrator.

The pharmacist shall be a member of the pharmaceutical services committee and the infection control committee. The pharmacist may be on other related committees.

The pharmacist shall report to the pharmaceutical services committee at least quarterly on the status of the facility's pharmaceutical services and staff performance. This report shall be made a part of the minutes of the committee. The pharmacist shall advise the pharmaceutical services committee of changes in drug laws and recommend methods of compliance. The pharmacist shall participate in drug utilization review.

The pharmacist shall be responsible for maintaining the contents of the emergency medication trays.

The pharmacist shall provide inservice education to the professional staffs on drugs and biologicals, including information on drug incompatibilities, new drugs, drug sensitivities, and drug interactions.

It is suggested that the pharmacist participate in patient/resident care conferences whenever possible.

### Standard III

A pharmaceutical services committee shall oversee the facility's pharmaceutical services, make recommendations for improvement, and monitor all drug-related services to assure accuracy.

The pharmaceutical services committee shall be composed of at least the pharmacist, administrator, medical director, and director of nursing. Other health professionals should be encouraged to be members of this committee. The committee shall meet at least quarterly and shall document its activities, findings, and recommendations.

The pharmaceutical services committee shall

- develop policies and procedures for the safe procurement, storage, distribution, use, and disposal of drugs and biologicals;
- establish procedures that prevent unauthorized drug usage and distribution, including procedures to account for the receipt and disposition of all drugs, particularly drugs subject to the Comprehensive Drug Abuse Prevention and Control Act of 1970;
- determine, in consultation with the medical staff and/or medical director, the contents of the emergency medication kit;
- determine which personnel are authorized to have access to keys to drug storage areas;
- develop, in consultation with the medical staff and/or medical director, a list of abbreviations and chemical symbols that are approved for use in ordering medications in the facility;
- establish, in consultation with the medical staff and/or medical director, stop-order policies to assure the appropriateness of continued drug therapy;
- determine what pharmaceutical reference materials should be available on the nursing units; and
- conduct ongoing drug utilization review.

The pharmaceutical services committee should also review the following.

- The formulary system, if one exists;
- Drug product recalls;
- Adverse drug reactions occurring within the facility; and
- All incidents involving medications.

## Standard IV

There shall be written policies and procedures governing the prescribing, storing, dispensing, administering, controlling, and disposing of all drugs and biologicals in compliance with all federal, state, and local laws and rules and regulations.

All medications for patients/residents shall be prescribed by a licensed physician or an individual allowed by state law to prescribe. All prescriptions are to be dispensed in accordance with written drug orders. All verbal drug orders shall be given to a licensed nurse, pharmacist, or physician. These orders shall be signed by the accepting person and countersigned by the attending physician within 48 hours.

The physician, pharmacist, and charge nurse shall review each patient's/resident's medications at least monthly or when there is a change in the patient's/resident's condition. When necessary, orders for medications shall be renewed by physician signature. A list of current medications shall be rewritten at least quarterly.

Automatic stop orders shall be placed on all medication orders that lack specific time or dosage limitations. The facility shall have written policies that specify when automatic stop orders on such medications become effective, and these policies shall be in compliance with all applicable federal, state, and local laws and rules and regulations. The attending physician shall be notified of the stop order prior to the last dose of a drug.

All drugs and biologicals shall be stored under proper conditions of temperature, light, and security. Medications shall be stored in a well-illuminated, locked storage device, cabinet, or room and shall be accessible only to authorized personnel. Medications being distributed shall be kept under continuous supervision. Medications for external use only shall be stored separately from internal medications and shall be accessible only to authorized personnel.

Schedule II controlled drugs subject to the Comprehensive Drug Abuse Prevention and Control Act of 1970 shall be stored in a cabinet of substantial construction under a double-lock system. If the facility uses the unit-dose system, the unit-dose cart may be under a single lock system.

The medications for each patient/resident shall be stored in original containers and shall not be transferred to other containers for storage. Each patient's/resident's medications shall be kept separate from others. With the exception of unit-dose packages, each original container shall be legibly marked with a securely attached label that clearly indicates the patient's/resident's full name; physician's name; prescription number; instructions for administration; date received; expiration date of all time-dated drugs; and name, address, and telephone number of pharmacy issuing the drug. In a unit-dose medication distribution system, each patient's/resident's supply of medications shall be stored in a container, bin, compartment, or drawer on which the patient's/resident's identity is clearly marked, and the prescriber's directions for drug administration shall be readily accessible. Labeling shall be in compliance with all currently accepted professional practices. When the manufacturer's lot or control number of medication is available, it is advisable to put it on the label. Medication containers that are damaged or poorly labeled shall be returned to the pharmacy for relabeling or disposal.

Pharmaceuticals requiring refrigeration shall be stored in a refrigerator located in a locked area, in a locked refrigerator, or in a separate locked and secured container within a refrigerator. The temperature in the refrigerator shall be checked at least monthly.

Drugs and biologicals shall be administered only by physicians, by licensed nursing personnel, or by other personnel who have satisfactorily completed a state-approved training program in medication administration. Drugs and biologicals are to be administered as soon as possible after doses are prepared and are to be administered by the same person who prepared the dose, except under unit-dose distribution systems. Each medication administered and the time of administration shall be promptly recorded in the patient's/resident's individual medication record and signed or initialed by the individual who administered the medication. In administering medications, medication cards or any other acceptable system shall be utilized and regularly checked against physician orders.

Medications prescribed for one patient/resident shall not be administered to any other patient/resident. Self administration of medications by patients/residents shall be permitted only when specifically authorized in writing by the attending physician. Control and supervision, however, is still the responsibility of the facility.

Medication errors and adverse drug reactions shall be reported to the patient's/resident's physician. If the situation is potentially life-threatening, it shall be reported immediately.

For control of Schedule II drugs subject to the Comprehensive Drug Abuse Prevention and Control Act of 1970, a separate record listing the following information shall be maintained for each substance, unless the facility uses a unit-dose distribution system.

- Substance.
- Prescription number.
- Amount received.
- Date received.
- Patient's/resident's name.
- Date and time administered.
- Dose.
- Physician's name.
- Signature of person administering drug.
- Balance remaining.

Records of controlled drugs are to be maintained in sufficient detail for accurate reconciliation. A count of narcotics shall be documented and signed at the end of each shift by the individual responsible.

There shall be written procedures for proper disposition of all medications and controlled drugs on the date of their expiration, upon discharge or death of a patient/resident, and upon discontinuation of medications and controlled drugs. These written procedures must assure full compliance with all existing federal, state, and local laws and rules and regulations.

A physician's written authorization shall be required for the release of prescription medications to patients/residents upon discharge. Each drug released shall be properly documented in the patient's/resident's record.

Medication reference material and up-to-date information shall be readily available.

# IV.  Standards of Practice for the Profession of Pharmacy

## Section I.  General Management and Administration of the Pharmacy

Selects and supervises pharmacists and nonprofessionals for pharmacy staff; establishes a pricing structure for pharmaceutical services and products; administers budgets and negotiates with vendors; develops and maintains a purchasing and inventory system for all drugs and pharmaceutical supplies; initiates a formulary system. In general, establishes and administers pharmacy management, personnel, and fiscal policy.

## Section II.  Activities Related To Processing the Prescription

Verifies prescription for legality and physical and chemical compatibility; checks patient record before dispensing prescription; measures quantities needed to dispense prescription; performs final check of finished prescription; dispenses prescriptions.

## Section III.  Patient Care Function

Clarifies patient's understanding of dosage; integrates drug-related with patient-related information; advises patient of potential drug-related conditions; refers patient to other health care resources; monitors and evaluates therapeutic response of patient; reviews and/or seeks additional drug-related information.

## Section IV.  Education of Health Care Professionals and Patients

Organizes, maintains, and provides drug information to other health care professionals; organizes and/or participates in "in-pharmacy" education programs for other pharmacists; makes recommendations regarding drug therapy to physician or patient; develops and maintains system for drug distribution and quality control.

# V.  Pharmaceutical Services in Skilled Nursing Facilities—The Intent of the Regulations (by Samuel W. Kidder, Pharm. D., M.P.H.)

## Introduction

Several years ago, the regulations dealing with Extended Care Facilities, commonly known as ECFs, began to undergo revision. This revision was initiated by the Department of Health, Education and Welfare to clarify certain requirements and update others so they more accurately reflected current practice and advancements in the nursing home industry. On January 17, 1974, the final regulations for Skilled Nursing Facilities (SNFs) were published in the *Federal Register*, and this paper explains the broad intent of these regulations.

This paper does not represent official HEW policy. This paper represents only the thinking of the author and is intended solely to provide the pharmacist with some initial guidance in endeavors to fulfill the requirements of the regulations.

Before beginning an explanation of the intent of the regulations, a few points should be made with respect to nomenclature, the process of regulation development, and the utility or purpose of these regulations.

The difference in terminology—ECFs vs. SNFs—is a result of Public Law 92—603 which requires uniform terminology and uniform regulations for nursing homes participating in either the Medicare or Medicaid programs. Prior to the enactment of Public Law 92—603, the Medicare program had regulations which it applied to nursing homes desiring participation in that program, and if a nursing home complied with these regulations it was termed an Extended Care Facility. In a similar manner, the Medicaid program had a separate set of regulations, and if a nursing home complied with these regulations it was termed a Skilled Nursing Home. (With respect to Pharmaceutical Services this is really a moot point—the regulations for these services were the same for both programs because Medicaid in the past had adopted Medicare's Pharmaceutical Services Condition of Participation by reference.) Congress, realizing that the two programs should have a uniform set of regulations with the same terminology, corrected this discrepancy by enacting Sections 246 and 278 of Public Law 92—603.

With respect to the process of regulation development, the regulations were first published as proposed rule-making which provided an opportunity for individuals and professional organizations (including the American Pharmaceutical Association and the American Society of Hospital Pharmacists) to comment. If the comments that resulted from the proposed rule-making publication were not incorporated in the final regulations, then the rationale for their rejections had to be justified and documented by the Department.

Regarding the utility or purpose of these regulations, it should be understood that it is very difficult to develop criteria for a particular aspect of health care delivery, promulgate them as regulations which becomes administrative law, and expect it to encompass every possible variation that can be found in thousands of health care facilities in 50 states and several territories.

However, if one views health care delivery in terms of structure, process, and outcome, these regulations deal primarily in structure and process (and do not attempt to measure outcome) and can be effectively used to measure the *capacity* of a facility to render quality care and, as such, are indirect measures of quality.

As Cashman and Myers (*Am. J. Public Health, 57,* July 1967) put it: "The key element here is that standards define a certain capacity for quality and not quality itself. We assume that given this capacity, a level of quality will result. And experience informs us that without this capacity, achievement of quality is difficult, if not impossible."

Thus, the assessment of quality health care cannot be truly attained by using these regulations as a measuring device. Quality health care has yet to be defined and indices for its measurement are yet to be refined. And once they are, they will be tools for practicing health care professionals to utilize in structures and processes such as Utilization Review Committees and Professional Standard Review Organizations.

The requirements pertaining to pharmaceutical services in these regulations are, for the most part, found in the three standards of the Nursing Services Condition of Participation and the four standards of the Pharmaceutical Services Condition of Participation. Before discussing the requirements found in these conditions, reference should be made to other requirements in the regulations that are of concern to pharmacists, although in some cases only indirectly.

# I. Definitions

In paragraph 405.1101 there are a number of definitions which are of importance to pharmacists.

1. *Approved Drugs and Biologicals*

**§405.1101 Definitions.**

As used in this subpart, the following definitions apply:

(b) *Approved drugs and biologicals.* Only such drugs and biologicals as are:
(1) In the case of Medicare:
(i) Included (or approved for inclusion) in the United States Pharmacopeia, National Formulary, or United States Homeopathic Pharmacopoeia; or
(ii) Included (or approved for inclusion) in AMA Drug Evaluations or Accepted Dental Therapeutics, except for any drugs and biologicals unfavorably evaluated therein; or
(iii) Not included (nor approved for inclusion) in the compendia listed in paragraphs (b)(1)(i) and (b)(1)(ii) of this section, may be considered approved if such drugs:
(A) Were furnished to the patient during his prior hospitalization, and
(B) Were approved for use during a prior hospitalization by the hospital's pharmacy and drug therapeutics committee (or equivalent), and
(C) Are required for the continuing treatment of the patient in the facility.
(2) In the case of Medicaid, those drugs approved by the State Title XIX agency.

With respect to Medicare this definition is almost word-for-word from the statute which relies on the various pharmaceutical compendia as the standard for drugs and biologicals paid for by Medicare. (See 1(i) and (ii)). Changing this regulation would require a change in the statute. Part of Medicare's definition of a drug and biological is new to the regulation (see 1(iii)(A)(B) and (C)), and states that some drugs which are not included or approved for inclusion may be considered approved if such drugs: were furnished to the patient during his or her prior hospitalization, were approved for use during a prior hospitalization by the hospital's pharmacy and therapeutics committee, and are required for the continuing treatment of the patient in the facility. This requirement allows reimbursement for a drug that is not in the compendium providing that *all three* criteria are met. That is, the patient must have been receiving the drug in the hospital, the drug must have been approved by the hospital's pharmacy and therapeutics committee, and the patient requires the drug for continuing treatment.

The definition of an approved drug and biological for the Medicaid program simply states that it be approved by the State Title XIX program leaving this determination entirely up to the State program.

Notice that this definition does *not* make reference to possibly or probably effective drugs. Separate regulations will be promulgated with respect to drugs classified as such and these regulations will cover all HEW programs that reimburse for drugs and biologicals and not simply drugs and biologicals utilized in Skilled Nursing Facilities under the Medicaid and Medicare programs.

### 2. *Controlled Drugs*

(d) *Controlled drugs.* Drugs listed as being subject to the Comprehensive Drug Abuse Prevention and Control Act of 1970 (Pub. L. 91—513) as set forth in 21 CFR Part 308.

Notice that this definition states that controlled drugs are drugs *listed as being* subject to the Comprehensive Drug Abuse Prevention and Control Act of 1970. This was written in this manner because all drugs are subject to this Act but only certain drugs are *listed* as controlled drugs.

### 3. *Drug Administration*

(h) *Drug administration.* An act in which a single dose of prescribed drug or biological is given to a patient by an authorized person in accordance with all laws and regulations governing such acts. The complete act of administration entails removing an individual dose from a previously dispensed, properly labeled container (including a unit dose container), verifying it with the physician's orders, giving the individual dose to the proper patient, and promptly recording the time and dose given.

It is important to notice that the definition stipulates that the complete act of administration entails the prompt recording of the time and dose given.

### 4. *Drug Dispensing*

(i) *Drug Dispensing.* An act entailing the interpretation of an order for a drug or biological and, pursuant to that order, the proper selection, measuring, labeling, packaging, and issuance of the drug or biological for a patient or for a service unit of the facility.

Notice that this definition provides for the issuance of the drug or biological to a patient or service unit of the facility. This allows the pharmacist to issue a drug or biological for a nursing service unit, as well as for a patient.

### 5. *Pharmacist*

(p) *Pharmacist.* A person who:
(1) Is licensed as a pharmacist by the State in which practicing, and
(2) Has training or experience in the specialized functions of institutional pharmacy, such as residencies in hospital pharmacy, seminars on institutional pharmacy, and related training programs.

This definition requires the pharmacist to be licensed, *and* trained *or* experienced in the specialized functions of institutional pharmacy. Therefore, a pharmacist to fulfill this requirement must be licensed and have either training *or* experience in institutional pharmacy.

The experience method of fulfilling the second portion of this requirement will probably be in terms of a specified number of years of experience in institutional pharmacy. Although it is yet to be determined, this experience will most likely be in terms of experience in a Medicare certified hospital or nursing home. A lesser number of years of full-time hospital experience will probably satisfy the requirement while a greater number of years as a part-time nursing home pharmacist will be necessary.

The training method of fulfilling the second portion of this requirement will in most cases be accomplished by seminars, workshops, etc. These instructional experiences will probably require about 20 hours of training with a specified number of hours being devoted to the various aspects of pharmaceutical services in nursing homes. For example, 1 hour on drug distribution systems, 2 hours on drug interactions, etc.

It is intended that the pharmacist serving the facility possess knowledge of the organization and the goals of the facility, how pharmaceutical services fit into that organization, and how these services contribute to the fulfillment of the facility's goals. In addition, the pharmacist should be familiar with the "state of the art" with respect to the delivery of pharmaceutical services to institutionalized patients. This, of course, means that the pharmacist should periodically update knowledge of institutional practice through continuing educational activities such as seminars and workshops. Even though some very objective criteria may be developed for this training or experience requirement, the overall guiding principle just stated should not be lost in understanding this requirement.

## II. Other Standards Important to the Pharmacist

1. *Paragraph 405.1121(e) Standard: Administrator.*

### §405.1121 Condition of participation— governing body and management.

The skilled nursing facility has an effective governing body, or designated persons so functioning, with full legal authority and responsibility for the operation of the facility. The governing body adopts and enforces rules and regulations relative to health care and safety of patients, to the protection of their personal and property rights, and to the general operation of the facility. The governing body develops a written institutional plan that reflects the operating budget and capital expenditures plan.

(e) *Standard: Administrator.* The governing body appoints a qualified administrator who is responsible for the overall management of the facility, enforces the rules and regulations relative to the level of health care and safety of patients, and to the protection of their personal and property rights, and plans, organizes, and directs those responsibilities delegated to him by the governing body. Through meetings and periodic reports, the administrator maintains ongoing liaison among the governing body, medical and nursing staffs, and other professional and supervisory staff of the facility, and studies and acts upon recommendations made by the utilization review and other committees. In the absence of the administrator, an employee is authorized, in writing, to act on his behalf.

Standard (e) of this condition of participation, among other things, requires the administrator to study and act on recommendations made by the utilization review and other committees. This is important to the pharmacist in that he or she is required to be a member of the Infection Control Committee and the Pharmaceutical Services Committee and could be a member of the Utilization Review Committee.

2. *Paragraph 405.1121(h) Standard: Staff Development.*

(h) *Standard: Staff Development.* An ongoing educational program is planned and conducted for the development and improvement of skills of all the facility's personnel, including training related to problems and needs of the aged, ill, and disabled. Each employee receives appropriate orientation to the facility and its policies, and to his position and duties. Inservice training includes at least prevention and control of infections, fire prevention and safety, accident prevention, confidentiality of patient information, and preservation of patient dignity, including protection of his privacy and personal and property rights. Records are maintained which indicate the content of, and attendance at, such staff development programs.

This standard requires that an ongoing educational program for the development and improvement of skills of *all* the facility's personnel be planned and conducted. This all inclusive requirement would include any inservice training the pharmacist could develop for nursing service personnel with respect to drug ordering, storage, distribution, administration, and monitoring.

3. *Paragraph 405.1121(i) Standard: Use of Outside Resources.*

(i) *Standard: Use of outside resources.* If the facility does not employ a qualified professional person to render a specific service to be provided by the facility, it makes arrangements to have such a service provided by an outside resource—a person or agency that will render direct service to patients or act as a consultant to the facility. The responsibilities, functions, and objectives, and the terms of agreement, including financial arrangements and charges, of each such outside resource are delineated in writing and signed by an authorized representative of the facility and the person or agency providing the service. Agreement pertaining to services must specify that the facility assumes professional and administrative responsibility for the services rendered. The outside resource, when acting as a consultant, apprises the administrator of recommendations, plans for implementation, and continuing assessment through dated, signed reports, which are retained by the administrator for followup action and evaluation of performance. (See requirement under each service—§§405.1125 through 405.1132.)

Standard (i) of this condition of participation requires that the description of the services of an outside resource be delineated in writing and be signed by a representative of the facility and the person providing the service. The agreement must specify that the facility assumes professional and administrative responsibility for the services rendered.

When the pharmacist serving the Skilled Nursing Facility is not a full-time employee of the facility, he or she will be considered an outside resource. Given the responsibilities placed on the pharmacist by these regulations, the pharmacist would be providing predominantly a direct service to patients and not acting as a consultant.

4. *Paragraph 405.1134(d) Standard: Nursing Unit.*

§405.1134 Condition of participation— Physical environment.

The skilled nursing facility is constructed, equipped, and maintained to protect the health and safety of patients, personnel, and the public.

(d) *Standard: Nursing unit.* Each nursing unit has at least the following basic service areas: Nurses station, storage and preparation area(s) for drugs and biologicals, and utility and storage rooms that are adequate in size, conveniently located, and well lighted to facilitate staff functioning. The nurses station is equipped to register patients' calls through a communication system from patient areas, including patient rooms and toilet and bathing facilities.

Standard (d) of the condition of participation contains certain requirements for the physical characteristics of drug storage and preparation areas. The determination of "adequate size," "conveniently located" and "well lighted" are left to the judgment of the surveyor. The obvious intent of this requirement is to preclude the use of a dark, cluttered, inaccessible area for drug preparation and storage, thereby, to the extent possible, prevent medication errors that may result from these factors. The regulation could have easily stated the number of square feet for storage and preparation areas, how many feet these areas must be from patient care areas, and how many foot candles of light must be present. However, rigid established criteria such as these frequently become the end, and not the means, and would not take into account variations in drug distribution systems presently in use today, or those that may be developed in the future.

5. *Paragraph 405.1135(a) Standard: Infection Control.*

### §405.1135 Condition of participation— infection control.

The skilled nursing facility establishes an infection control committee of representative professional staff responsible for overall infection control in the facility. All necessary housekeeping and maintenance services are provided to maintain a sanitary and comfortable environment and to help prevent the development and transmission of infection.

(a) *Standard: Infection control committee.* The infection control committee is composed of members of the medical and nursing staffs, administration, and dietetic, pharmacy, housekeeping, maintenance, and other services; the committee establishes policies and procedures for investigating, controlling, and preventing infections in the facility, and monitors staff performance to ensure that the policies and procedures are executed.

Standard (a) of the condition of participation requires that an Infection Control Committee be established and the pharmacist be a member of that committee. The intent of having the pharmacist a member of this committee stems from a need for expertise with respect to the efficacy of various antiseptics and germicides used in the facility. It also could capitalize on his or her expertise with regard to the indiscriminate use of antibiotics, although this is a function that may be more appropriately handled by the Utilization Review Committee.

6. *Paragraph 405.1137(c) Standard: Medical Care Evaluation Studies.*

### §405.1137 Condition of participation— utilization review.

The skilled nursing facility carries out review of the services provided in the facility at least to inpatients who are entitled to benefits under the program(s). Utilization review has as its overall objectives both the maintenance of high quality patient care and assurance of appropriate and efficient utilization of facility services. There are two elements to utilization review: medical care evaluation studies that identify and examine patterns of care provided in the facility, and review of extended duration cases which is concerned with efficiency, appropriateness, and cost effectiveness of care. If the Secretary determines that the utilization review procedures established pursuant to title XIX are superior in their effectiveness to the procedures required under this section, he may, to the extent that he deems it appropriate, require for purposes of this title that the procedures established pursuant to title XIX be utilized instead of the procedures required by this section.

(c) *Standard: Medical care evaluation studies.* Medical care evaluation studies are performed to promote the most effective and appropriate use of available health facilities and services consistent with patient needs and professionally recognized standards of health care. Studies, which could include assessment of findings resulting from periodic medical review, emphasize identification and analysis of patterns of patient care and changes indicated to maintain consistent high quality of services. Each medical care evaluation study (whether medical or administrative in emphasis) identifies and analyzes factors related to the patient care rendered in the facility, and serves as the basis for recommendations for change beneficial to patients, staff, the facility, and the community. Studies on a sample or other basis, include but need not be limited to, admissions, durations of stay, and professional services (including drugs and biologicals) furnished. At least one study is in progress at any given time.

Paragraph 405.1137 requires the establishment of a Utilization Review Committee which is composed of two or more physicians and optionally other professional personnel. Utilization review has as its overall objective both the maintenance of high quality patient care and the appropriate and efficient utilization of the facility's services. Standard (c) of this condition of participation requires that medical care evaluation studies be performed and that these studies include but need not be limited to admissions, durations of stay, and professional services (including drugs and biologicals) furnished.

By virtue of training and experience, the pharmacist is in a unique position to develop and implement studies of professional services that deal with drugs and biologicals. The pharmacist's expertise can be used to improve the use of drugs in Skilled Nursing Facilities through this study requirement.

HEW had a contract with the University of Minnesota School of Pharmacy for the development of model studies for 10 different drugs commonly used in Skilled Nursing Facilities. Pharmacists can use these model studies or adopt them for use in complying with the intent of this requirement which, in the case of drugs and biologicals, is to improve the chemotherapeutic care of the skilled nursing facility patient.

## III. Pharmacy Requirements of the Nursing Services Condition of Participation

The Nursing Services Condition of Participation contains three standards that deal with pharmaceutical services:

1. *Paragraph 405.1124(g) Standard: Administration of Drugs*

### §405.1124 Condition of participation— nursing services.

The skilled nursing facility provides 24-hour service by licensed nurses, including the services of a registered nurse at least during the day tour of duty 5 days a week. There is an organized nursing service with a sufficient number of qualified nursing personnel to meet the total nursing needs of all patients.

(g) *Standard: Administration of drugs.* Drugs and biologicals are administered only by physicians, licensed nursing personnel, or by other personnel who have completed a State-approved training program in medication administration. Procedures are established by the pharmaceutical services committee (see §405.1127(d)) to ensure that drugs to be administered are checked against physician's orders, that the patient is identified prior to administration of a drug, and that each patient has an individual medication record and that the dose of drug administered to that patient is properly recorded therein by the person who administered the drug. Drugs and biologicals are administered as soon as possible after doses are prepared, and are administered by the same person who prepared the doses for administration, except under single unit dose package distribution systems. (See §405.1101(h).)

Standard (g) of the condition of participation has a number of requirements in narrative form which must be separated out for discussion:

a. The requirement dealing with who may administer a drug and biological is restricted to physicians, licensed nurses, and individuals who have completed a state-approved program in drug administration.

The intent of allowing other than physicians and licensed nursing personnel (RNs, LVNs, LPNs) to administer drugs is to free nursing personnel to provide more skilled nursing services. At the same time this requirement provides some assurance that those individuals who may assume this task have sufficient training so as not to jeopardize the health and safety of the patient. By virtue of their present professional training and experience, licensed nursing personnel will be deemed to meet this requirement.

Whether or not a program will be approved by the State is up to the State and this regulation does not force states into offering such programs or approving such programs. Moreover, if a State's Nurse Practice Act precludes unlicensed personnel from performing

the act of drug administration then the State's Nurse Practice Act will prevail.

b. This standard also has a requirement for the maintenance of an individual medication record and that the dose of drug administered to the patient is properly recorded therein by the person who administers the drug. The intent of the individual medication record is two fold. First, it is required so that the pharmacist has a single complete record of all drugs a particular patient is using so that the monthly review of the patient's medication record can be performed. (This review will be discussed later.) Secondly, this record could be designed so that the receipt and disposition of all controlled drugs could be maintained. The rationale for the second purpose is to reduce the number of records that must be maintained by the facility. It is hoped that one record may suffice for both the performance of the review of the patient's drug regimen and the maintenance of a record for the receipt and disposition of controlled drugs. On a practical basis, this two fold purpose may not be accomplished by a single record, but the facility and the pharmacist will have the flexibility to reduce their recordkeeping through this mechanism.

c. This standard also requires that drugs and biologicals:

(1) be administered by the same person who prepares them for administration (pours meds),

(2) be promptly recorded by the same person who administers them, and

(3) be administered as soon as possible after preparation for administration.

The combined intent of these criteria is to provide continuity in drug administration which reduces the probability that drug administration errors will occur. The intent of (3) above is to preclude the preparation of drugs for administration for more than one shift at a time thereby precluding, to the extent possible, the contamination or deterioration of liquid dosage forms, or accidentally spilling solid dosage forms and returning them to a receptacle designated for another patient. Number (1) above also fulfills this intent because it is unlikely that the person preparing drugs for administration will be working two consecutive shifts, thus, enabling the same individual to prepare drugs during one shift and administering them during the next shift.

The exception for single unit dose-package distribution systems (unit doses) was included in this standard because the act of preparing drugs for administration, in these systems, occurs during the act of drug dispensing and the chances for contamination, deterioration, and spillage are remote.

2. *Paragraph 405.1124(h) Standard: Conformance with Physicians' Drug Orders.*

(h) *Standard: Conformance with physicians' drug orders.* Drugs are administered in accordance with written orders of the attending physician. Drugs not specifically limited as to time or number of doses when ordered are controlled by automatic stop orders or other methods in accordance with written policies. Physicians' verbal orders for drugs are given only to a licensed nurse, pharmacist, or physician and are immediately recorded and signed by the person receiving the order. (Verbal orders for Schedule II drugs are permitted only in the case of a bona fide emergency situation.) Such orders are countersigned by the attending physician within 48 hours. The attending physician is notified of an automatic stop order prior to the last dosage so that he may decide if the administration of the drug or biological is to be continued or altered.

The first statement in this standard simply requires that drugs be administered upon the order of the physician. This order does not always have to be in writing since there is provision for receipt of a physician's verbal order providing that such orders are countersigned within 48 hours. The second statement in this standard deals with stop order policies and its intent is to prevent the receipt of drugs by the patient beyond the period of time that the drug is medically necessary. The facility may wish to adopt certain stop order policies to fulfill the intent of this requirement, or it may develop "other methods" to fulfill the intent of this requirement. The establishment of stop order policies which require professional discretion should be established by the professional staff of the facility. However, if stop order policies are obviously unrealistic, then the facility will not be fulfilling the intent of this requirement.

The statement pertaining to who may receive a physician's verbal order includes another physician, pharmacist, or licensed nurse. The pharmacist was added to this criterion because pharmacists receive verbal drug orders routinely while serving outpatients and should not be precluded from doing so for skilled nursing facility patients. The problem encountered with this practice occurs when nursing personnel receive the completed order and are reluctant to administer the drug in the absence of knowledge that the physician ever ordered it. However, this problem is reduced by the requirement for countersigning verbal orders within 48 hours which would give nursing personnel the validation they seek.

3. *Paragraph 405.1124(i) Standard: Storage of Drugs and Biologicals.*

(i) *Standard: Storage of drugs and biologicals.* Procedures for storing and disposing of drugs and biologicals are established by the pharmaceutical services committee. In accordance with State and Federal laws, all drugs and biologicals, are stored in locked compartments under proper temperature controls and only authorized personnel have access to the keys. Separately locked, permanently affixed compartments are provided for storage of controlled drugs listed in Schedule II of the Comprehensive Drug Abuse Prevention & Control Act of 1970 and other drugs subject to abuse, except under single unit package drug distribution systems in which the quantity stored is minimal and a missing dose can be readily detected. An emergency medication kit approved by the pharmaceutical services committee is kept readily available.

This standard requires that all drugs be locked and that Schedule II drugs by separately locked. The obvious intent of these provisions is to protect drugs stored in the facility from unauthorized use. The term separately locked means that the key used to gain access to non-Schedule II drugs is not the same key used to gain access to the Schedule II drugs. (Obviously these keys cannot be on the same ring or holder.) The authorized personnel who have access to the keys is to be determined by the Pharmaceutical Services Committee.

The separately locked requirement for "other drugs subject to abuse" was included in the event the facility felt that non-Schedule II drugs were being abused and wished to provide better security for them. The determination as to what other drugs may be subject for abuse is left up to the facility's Pharmaceutical Services Committee.

The term "compartment" as it is used in this standard includes, but is not limited to: rooms, drawers, cabinets, carts, refrigerators, and boxes. The exception from the "separately locked" provision for single unit package drug distribution systems (unit dose) was necessary so the development of this type of drug distribution system would not be inhibited. However, this exception may only be granted if all three criteria are met. The system must in fact be a unit dose system and not simply a supply of drugs individually wrapped. The quantity stored must be minimal (e.g., a 24—48-hour supply) and a missing dose must be readily detected. In interpreting this requirement it must be remembered that Schedule II drugs in a unit dose drug distribution system are only exempt from the separately locked provision and are not exempted from the requirement that all drugs be locked. The exemption for unit dose merely allows Schedule II drugs in unit dose systems to be stored and locked with other drugs and not separately stored and locked. The criterion as to whether a missing dose can be readily detected should be based on the amount of time it takes to make the determination—generally not more than a few minutes.

The last requirement of this standard deals with an emergency medication kit. This standard only requires that this kit be available. The contents of this kit are left to the professional discretion of the Pharmaceutical Services Committee within the constraints of State and local laws. This kit should be sealed, but it should not be locked. It must, as all drugs, be stored in a locked compartment. The determination as to the ready availability of the emergency medication kit should be made by an assessment of its contents and how urgently the contents may be needed. If the kit contains drugs used in cardiac or respiratory arrest, the kit must be more readily available than if it contained only analgesics or tranquilizers. The kit should have a diagram showing its contents and should be checked by the pharmacist during regularly scheduled visits.

## IV. Requirements of the Pharmaceutical Services Condition of Participation

1. *Paragraph 405.1127 Condition of Participation —Pharmaceutical Services.*

### §405.1127 Condition of participation— pharmaceutical services.

The skilled nursing facility provides appropriate methods and procedures for the dispensing and administering of drugs and biologicals. Whether drugs and biologicals are obtained from the community or institutional pharmacists or stocked by the facility, the facility is responsible for providing such drugs and biologicals for its patients, insofar as they are covered under the programs, and for ensuring that pharmaceutical services are provided in accordance with accepted professional principles and appropriate Federal, State, and local laws. (See §405.1124(g), (h), and (i).)

The Pharmaceutical Services Condition of Participation defines in broad terms the responsibility of the facility to provide these services to its patients, and it requires that these services be provided in accordance with accepted professional principles which are defined in the four standards of this condition of participation and the three standards in the Nursing Services Condition of Participation previously described. The Pharmaceutical Services Condition of Participation also allows the facility the latitude of maintaining its own pharmacy or obtaining its drugs and biologicals from a community or institutional pharmacy.

2. *Paragraph 405.1127(a) Standard: Supervision of Services.*

(a) *Standard: Supervision of services.* The pharmaceutical services are under the general supervision of a qualified pharmacist who is responsible to the administrative staff for developing, coordinating, and supervising all pharmaceutical services. The pharmacist (if not a full-time employee) devotes a sufficient number of hours, based upon the needs of the facility, during regularly scheduled visits to carry out these responsibilities. The pharmacist reviews the drug regimen of each patient at least monthly, and reports any irregularities to the medical director and administrator. The pharmacist submits a written report at least quarterly to the pharmaceutical services committee on the status of the facility's pharmaceutical service and staff performance.

This standard has been changed significantly in that the concept of consultant pharmacist has been deleted in favor of defining a staff responsibility for the pharmacist. Experience in the Medicare program has demonstrated that the consultant concept as applied to the pharmaceutical services was insufficient. In many facilities, pharmacists have provided good phar-

maceutical services, but in the majority, the pharmacist was only a "paper consultant" who merely lent name and license number to the facility. This staff responsibility is defined by making the pharmacist responsible to the administrator for developing, coordinating, and supervising *all* pharmaceutical services. Whether or not the term "consultant" is used to describe the pharmacist who serves the facility is immaterial. The important thing is that the concept be deleted and the role for the pharmacist that is denoted by the term "consultant" be deleted.

The term "responsible" in this standard means that the pharmacist is broadly responsible for all pharmaceutical services in the facility. He or she has joint responsibility with the nursing service in all aspects of drug ordering, storage, distribution, administration, and charting. (See 405.1125, Standards (g), (h), and (i).) In addition to the specific areas of responsibility set forth in the Pharmaceutical Services Condition, the pharmacist is responsible for determining that:

(i) Policies and procedures are being followed.
(ii) No discontinued, outdated, deteriorated, or recalled drugs or biologicals are available for use in the facility.
(iii) Drug containers with illegible, incomplete, makeshift, damaged, worn, soiled, or missing labels are returned to the dispensing pharmacist for disposition.
(iv) Drugs for external use and poisons are kept separate from other medications.
(v) Patients' medication records are accurate and up to date.
(vi) Antiseptics, disinfectants, and germicides used in patient care have legible, distinctive labels that identify the contents and include instruction for use.
(vii) Compartments containing drugs and biologicals are locked when not in use, and trays and carts used to transport drugs are not left unattended.

The responsibilities described above, those described in the other standards of this Condition, and others the facility and the pharmacist may mutually deem appropriate, should be delineated in a written job description which is legally consummated by a written agreement. The written agreement should describe the financial arrangements between the pharmacist and the facility concerning payment for: (1) the pharmaceutical service provided by the pharmacist, and (2) the drug products provided by the pharmacist. (See paragraph 405.1121(i) Standard: Use of Outside Resources, for more discussion of this written agreement.)

The "sufficient number of hours" requirement in this standard is a variable criterion, and compliance with this criterion depends on the size and scope of the service, the type of drug distribution system employed, and a number of other variables. In some facilities the pharmacist may only have to serve a few hours a week, but in others it may require full-time employment. In some facilities, it initially may require a considerable amount of time for the pharmacist to develop and implement a safe, efficient, and controlled drug distribution system, but subsequently it may require only a portion of that initial time.

The pharmacist must devote a sufficient number of hours during a regularly scheduled visit. The frequency of this visit should be consistent with the needs of the facility and will vary depending on those needs. To fulfill the responsibilities defined in these regulations, the frequency of these visits should generally be weekly conscientiously.

The pharmacist's review of the drug regimen of each patient in the facility at least monthly is a positive effort to reduce drug interactions, duplications, and medication errors. By making a single qualified health professional, who specializes in this area of patient care, responsible for this review, the incidence of chemotherapeutic errors and overutilization can be demonstrably reduced. When the pharmacist determines, through a review of the patient's drug regimen, that there is a potential problem, he or she should report this to the medical director and the administrator, and if the situation warrants it, to the utilization review committee. If the problem the pharmacist discovers deals with inappropriate drug administration, these findings should be reported to the director of nursing, and if the situation warrants it to the medical director and the administrator. The intent of this requirement is primarily to improve the quality of chemotherapeutic care to patients in skilled nursing facilities, and secondarily to reduce the cost of this care.

The question as to *where* the pharmacist must perform this drug regimen review is important. Good arguments can be made for the performance of this review in the pharmacy, thus enabling the pharmacist to detect any drug interactions or adverse reactions before dispensing the drug.

An equally good argument can be made for the performance of this review in the facility, thus enabling the pharmacist to be familiar with the patient, the diagnosis or diagnoses, dietary requirements, and the results of any laboratory work that may be performed. However, since this is a new responsibility for the pharmacist, it may be advisable to gradually phase into this activity by performing this review in the pharmacy, and gaining the necessary familiarity with the patient during regularly scheduled visits to the facility. The highest order of fulfilling this requirement would be for the pharmacist to perform this task in the facility.

For the state agency surveyor to determine that the facility has complied with this requirement, there must be some documentation showing that the pharmacist has performed a review of each patient's drug regimen. The question as to where this documentation should be maintained is important. If it becomes a permanent part of the patient's medical record, it cannot contain any opinions that require medical judgment. (The regulations (see 405.1132(d)) only allow the physician to enter or authenticate into the medical record opinions that require medical judgment.) Thus, if the pharmacist chooses to maintain this documentation in the medical record he or she would be restricted to facts and could not express opinions. For example, the pharmacist could state that the patient was receiving chlorpromazine 50 mg three times a day and thioridazine 10 mg four times a day but could not say that these two drugs were the reason that the patient was so lethargic—the latter represents an opinion that requires medical judgment. The pharmacist could also enter into the permanent medical record that the patient's drug regimen was reviewed but could not state in that record that any drug irregularities were found because that also represents an opinion that requires medical judgment.

A means to overcome this restriction would be to arrange for the pharmacist's report to not become a *permanent* part of the medical record. This may allow the pharmacist to record opinions that require medical judgments. Whether or not this method could be used is dependent on the facilities' policies with respect to the contents of the permanent medical record.

Another means to resolve the problem would be the maintenance of a separate record for drug regimen review summaries. This separate record would allow the pharmacist to enter appropriate opinions. It would provide the surveyor with the documentation to determine if the requirement has been fulfilled. Since the pharmacist must report drug irregularities to the medical director and the administrator who are responsible for informing the attending physician, it is not imperative to bring drug irregularities to the attention of the attending physician via the medical record. In some cases, it may not even be advisable for the pharmacist's report to be contained in the medical record since it is possible for the report to become lost or obscured among all the other documents contained in the medical record. The important thing to remember is that a review be performed and that, if clinically significant irregularities are detected pursuant to that review, the attending physician is informed. Whether the physician is informed by means of the medical record or a drug regimen review summary is not as important as seeing to it that he or she is informed of a potentially hazardous situation that involves the drug(s) that are being administered to the patient.

The intent of the requirement that the pharmacist report drug irregularities to the medical director and the administrator rather than to the attending physician is based on the premise that the medical director would probably have better rapport with the attending physician than the pharmacist. Obviously, this may not be true in all circumstances, and the regulations do not preclude the pharmacist from reporting irregularities to the attending physician as well as the medical director and administrator. The intent of the requirement is to improve the chemotherapeutic care of the patient, and the pharmacist should not feel constrained by the reporting scheme described in these regulations if it is more realistic to simply report findings to the attending physician. But in doing so the pharmacist should also inform the medical director of the findings and of the direct report to the attending physician. Moreover, the pharmacist should not neglect to report findings to the administrator because he or she is the facility's liaison between the professional staff and the governing body which is ultimately responsible for the services rendered by the facility. (See 405.1121(e) Standard: Administrator and 405.1121(i) Standard: Use of Outside Resources.)

The requirement that the pharmacist submit a written report at least quarterly is necessary to have a professional analysis of the total system for delivery of pharmaceutical services in the facility and based upon this analysis, formulates rational comprehensive recommendations aimed at the improvement of these services. This written report serves the administrator by providing professional advice and by presenting various management options that he or she could pursue with respect to the provision of quality pharmaceutical services. The report should also be submitted to the Pharmaceutical Services Committee to assist this Committee to fulfill its responsibility as an overseer of pharmaceutical services in the facility.

3. *Paragraph 405.1127(b) Control and Accountability.*

(b) *Standard: Control and Accountability.* The pharmaceutical service has procedures for control and accountability of all drugs and biologicals throughout the facility. Only approved drugs and biologicals are used in the facility, and are dispensed in compliance with Federal and State laws. Records of receipt and disposition of all controlled drugs are maintained in sufficient detail to enable an accurate reconciliation. The pharmacist determines that drug records are in order and that an account of all controlled drugs is maintained and reconciled.

The pharmacist's responsibility with respect to control and accountability is stressed in this standard. The intent of this requirement is that the Pharmaceutical Services Committee establish procedures that prevent the unauthorized use of drugs and biologicals. This will require the establishment of procedures that will provide for an accounting of the receipt and disposition of all drugs, and in particular, drugs subject to the Comprehensive Drug Abuse Prevention and Control Act of 1970.

The intent of this standard is not to be construed to mean that excessive and time-consuming records must be kept to account for over-the-counter drugs such as aspirin or milk of magnesia, but rather to account for drugs which can only be legally prescribed by a physician, and especially those which are subject to abuse.

The pharmacist has the responsibility of determining during regularly scheduled visits whether or not an account of all controlled drugs is being maintained and reconciled. This means that the pharmacist must determine if records are being kept up to date and whether the number of controlled drugs received corresponds with the number of drugs administered and the number remaining. If discrepancies occur, it is the pharmacist's responsibility to alert the director of nursing so that more stringent control procedures can be instituted. The intent of the requirement is not to be construed to mean that the nursing personnel must perform a reconciliation of controlled drugs at the end of each tour of duty, or for that matter, on a daily basis. This is a waste of valuable nursing time that should be devoted to nursing care. The intent is, however, to provide for a record of controlled drugs by which, at any point in time, one could determine if these drugs were being improperly channeled. If they were being improperly channeled, then a reconciliation may be necessary on a daily basis or after each tour of duty.

In most cases, the individual medication record (see 405.1125(g)) can be used to fulfill this requirement for drugs distributed through the individual prescription and unit dose systems. If floor stocks of legend drugs are permitted by State law, then individual medication records would not be practical, and in order to fulfill this requirement, a separate record of the receipt and disposition of drugs maintained under this system would be required. This is especially applicable to drugs subject to the Comprehensive Drug Abuse

Prevention and Control Act of 1970.

The requirement that only approved drugs and biologicals are used in the facility relates back to the legal definitions of a drug and a biological (see Definitions 405.1101).

The requirement stating that drugs are dispensed in compliance with Federal and State laws defers the question of who may dispense drugs to the appropriate State laws and regulations dealing with the performance of this act. In general this means that: Only the pharmacist, or authorized pharmacy personnel under the direct supervision of the pharmacist, compounds or dispenses drugs and biologicals, prepares, labels, or makes labeling changes, and that when the pharmacist is not available, drugs are removed from the pharmacy (or drug storage area) only by a designated licensed nurse or a physician, and only in amounts sufficient for immediate therapeutic needs, and a record is maintained of such withdrawals.

4. *Paragraph 405.1127(c) Standard: Labeling of Drugs and Biologicals.*

(c) *Standard: Labeling of drugs and biologicals.* The labeling of drugs and biologicals is based on currently accepted professional principles, and includes the appropriate accessory and cautionary instructions, as well as the expiration date when applicable.

In earlier drafts of this standard specific information was required to be on the label of a prescription container. However, it became apparent that different drug distribution systems required different labeling information. It also became apparent that specific labeling requirements promulgated as regulations resulted in a great deal of inflexibility. Therefore, it was determined that the requirement would simply read that labeling would be in accordance with accepted professional principles, and these accepted professional principles would be defined in the interpretative guidelines. This would allow for easier changes in the specific labeling requirements as accepted professional principles change.

The labeling requirements for each drug distribution system are as follows:

1. The label of each patient's individual drug container bears the full name; the prescribing physician's name; and the name, strength, and quantity of the drug dispensed. Appropriate accessory and cautionary statements are included, as well as the expiration date when applicable. The quantity of drug dispensed is required on this label so as to facilitate the record of receipt and disposition of drug and especially Schedule II drugs.

2. The label of each floor stock drug container bears the name and strength of the drug, lot and control number, expiration date when applicable, and any other appropriate accessory or cautionary statement.

3. Each single unit package bears the name and strength of the drug and the lot or control number and is clearly identified with the patient's full name and the prescribing physician's name. Appropriate accessory and cautionary statements are included, as well as the expiration date when applicable. The clearly identified single unit package labeling requirement means that the name of the patient and the physician do not have to be on the label of the package, but the name of the patient and the physician must be identified with the package in such a manner as to *assure* that the drug is administered to the right patient.

4. The labeling requirements of over-the-counter drugs (drugs which do not legally require a prescription) is based on criteria established by the Pharmaceutical Services Committee.

*5. Paragraph 405.1127(d) Standard: Pharmaceutical Services Committee.*

(d) *Standard: Pharmaceutical services committee.* A pharmaceutical services committee (or its equivalent) develops written policies and procedures for safe and effective drug therapy, distribution, control, and use. The committee is comprised of at least the pharmacist, the director of nursing services, the administrator, and one physician. The committee oversees pharmaceutical service in the facility, makes recommendations for improvement, and monitors the service to ensure its accuracy and adequacy. The committee meets at least quarterly and documents its activities, findings, and recommendations.

The Pharmaceutical Services Committee is necessary because there is a great need to coordinate the various professionals involved in the provision of this service. With increasing reliance on chemotherapy, it is important that a multidisciplinary committee such as this develop and monitor sound policies for drug distribution, control and use. The committee is comprised of at least the pharmacist, the director of nursing, the administrator, and one physician.

This standard clearly establishes the facility's Pharmaceutical Services Committee as the body responsible for the development of policies and procedures dealing with pharmaceutical services. The pharmacist serving the facility is responsible for authoritative guidance in developing these policies and procedures.

The Pharmaceutical Services Committee should specifically:

1. Receive and appropriately act on the pharmacist's written report (see 405.1127(a)).

2. Establish stop-order policies or other methods to assure the appropriateness of continued drug therapy (see 415.1124(h)).

3. Determines the contents of the emergency medication kit (see 405.1124(i)). The contents of the emergency medication kit must be in compliance with State laws and regulations.

4. Develops a list of abbreviations and chemical symbols that are approved for use in ordering medications in the facility.

5. Develops policies and procedures for the safe

procurement, storage, distribution, and use of drugs and biologicals (see 405.1124(i)).

6. Determines which personnel will be authorized to have access to the keys to the drug storage area (see 405.1124(i)).

7. Determine labeling requirements for over-the-counter drugs.

8. Establish policies for the use of drugs brought to the facility by the patient.

# VI. Saving Cost, Quality and People: Drug Reviews in Long-Term Care, By Samuel W. Kidder, reprinted from *American Pharmacy,* NS18, 346(1978).

The Medicare and Medicaid regulation that requires a pharmacist to review monthly the drug regimen of each skilled nursing facility patient has the potential for savings in these programs of $3.2 to $37.2 million a year.

These savings are *in addition to* those that could accrue from the prevention of inappropriate drug therapy, such as a reduction in unnecessary hospitalization. Furthermore, such savings can be achieved while enhancing the quality of drug therapy. Before examining the savings and quality improvement potential of monthly drug review in skilled nursing facilities, a discussion of the important events that led to the present situation is in order.

## Paradox: Clinical Pharmacists, Paper Consultants and Drug Problems

Before the enactment of Medicare, pharmacists had been involved in providing services to nursing homes, but this, in the words of one editor, "consisted primarily of delivering to the home a large bottle of aspirin or a dozen bottles of milk of magnesia and the occasional dispensing of presciption medication for an unseen nursing home patient."[1]

The extended care facility regulations published pursuant to Title XVIII of the Social Security Amendments of 1965 to a large extent codified existing practice standards[a] and required pharmacists actively to engage in consultation covering procurement, storage, selection, packaging, distribution and administration of drugs and biologicals. These services are usually referred to as "consultant pharmacist" services and they involve the nondispensing services pharmacists carry out for these facilities.

The extended care facility regulations were enthusiastically greeted by pharmacists. This journal devoted the entire May 1966 issue to the subject, encouraging pharmacists to become involved in this type of service. Pharmacists by and large accepted the challenge, began actively to provide consultant services, and were—to a demonstrable degree—compensated for their services.

In a 1968 study by McLeod and Eckel,[2] 58 percent of the pharmacists serving 38 nursing homes were doing an acceptable job of providing consultant services. Of this group, 63 percent were being compensated. In 1969, even this barely optimal picture began to change. In April of that year the Medicare Program began to restrict reimbursement, consistent with congressional intent, for extended care benefits. Between 1969 and 1970, Medicare reimbursement for these benefits dropped 33 percent.[3] This and a subsequent increase, then leveling, then decline[4] in Medicaid reimbursement for skilled nursing care did a lot to drive consultants back to their pharmacies, thus contributing substantially to the development of the "paper consultant" phenomenon in which the pharmacist-consultant of record seldom did more than supply "prescription medication to unseen nursing home patients." The return of consultants to their pharmacies and the "paper consultant" phenomenon is evidenced by data from a limited study indicating that 75 percent of nursing home patients did not receive adequate pharmaceutical services and drug control.[5]

Meanwhile, in the early seventies reports of "overdrugging" and "medication errors" in nursing homes began to leak out into the lay, professional and congressional press. [6] [7] [8] [9] In 1970 hearings before the Subcommittee on Long-Term Care of the Senate Special Committee on Aging mentioned the problem of the improper use of tranquilizers.[10] A 1970 General Accounting Office audit entitled "Continuing Problems of Providing Nursing Home Care and Prescribed Drugs under the Medicaid Program in California" showed—in a review of one month's medical records of 106 Medicaid patients at 14 nursing homes—that 311 doses were administered in quantities in excess of those prescribed, and 1,210 prescribed doses were not administered.[11]

Considerable public attention was also focused on the problem by Senator Frank Moss, the former chairman of the Subcommittee on Long-Term Care. This attention culminated in a January 1975 report[12] which discusses, among other items, problems of medication errors, adverse drug reactions, drug addiction, and "chemical straight jackets." The recommendations of this report implicitly called for greater pharmacist involvement in the supervision and provision of pharmaceutical services in nursing homes.

A concurrent development was the considerable interest generated during the late sixties over the so-called "clinical pharmacist." This interest resulted in the convening of the Task Force on the Pharmacist's Clinical Role, which was charged with the responsibility of "the development of a set of working criteria for a clinical role." The work of the task force was published in September 1971.[13] Although the task force report did not specifically mention long-term care facilities as a setting in which clinical pharmacy could be practiced, it did list a number of functions which could be applied to this setting.

In 1970 the Bureau of Health Manpower of the Department of Health, Education and Welfare's (HEW's) Health Resources Administration, began increasing its support of pharmacy schools and students, pursuant to the Health Manpower Act of 1968. This support, which has amounted to more than $185 million[14] between fiscal years 1970 and 1976, has been used to a substantial degree to prepare pharmacists for clinically oriented services such as patient drug regimen reviews. Such reviews could substantially ameliorate demonstrated drug problems in nursing homes.

## Proscribing the Paradox

The "paper consultant" phenomenon, the training of "clinical pharmacists," the problems of "overdrugging" in nursing homes—all influenced the development of skilled nursing facility regulations of 1974.[15] These regulations significantly expanded pharmacist involvement in skilled nursing facilities by making this health professional "responsible to the administrative staff for developing, coordinating and supervising all pharmaceutical services." In a specific effort to solve the problem of inappropriate drug therapy, the regulations required the pharmacist to review "the drug regimen of each patient at least monthly and report any irregularities to the medical director and administrator."

The responsibilities of consultant pharmacists were therefore strengthened and expanded beyond the consultative role defined by the original regulations. The new regulations not only increased the pharmacist's responsibility for *all* pharmaceutical services, but added a significant new drug monitoring responsibility in the form of a monthly drug regimen review of each patient. This latter function shifted the emphasis of pharmaceutical services in these facilities from consultation on the manipulation and storage of drug products to a staff responsibility for monitoring the patients' response to drug therapy.[b]

Requiring greater pharmacy consultation and drug monitoring services—with emphasis on the patient—was a logical response to the significant drug therapy problems that existed in skilled and other nursing facilities. The regulations offered pharmacists an opportunity to use their clinical drug monitoring skills and improve the drug therapy of skilled nursing facility patients. Such monitoring also gave the public a greater return on the investment their tax dollars were making to pharmacy schools through the Health Manpower Act of 1968.

## Implementing the SNF Regulations

HEW began implementing the regulations by providing state survey and certification agencies with interpretive guidelines and survey procedures. Public Law 93-368 authorized surveyor training programs which allowed 100 percent federal funding of salaries and training of surveyors in long-term care. [16] In addition, training for long-term care facility staff was begun through contracts let by the Division of Long Term Care of HEW's Health Resources Administration. One of these contracts[17] was specifically aimed at training pharmacists for service in the nursing home setting and especially for monitoring drug therapy in skilled nursing facilities.

In July 1975, HEW released the Introductory Report of the Long Term Care Facility Improvement Study. This study showed that approximately eight months after the regulations became effective, 68 percent of the pharmacists serving skilled nursing facilities were reviewing the drug regimens of patients at least monthly.[18] This level of compliance is probably acceptable given that only eight months had passed since the regulations had become final.

However, the same report showed that 66 percent of the pharmacists spent less than five hours per week in the facility, and that 86 percent of the drug profile records were located at places other than the skilled nursing facility. In order to perform in-depth reviews,

In October 1975, the Medicare program released its "Provider Reimbursement Manual" revision dealing with costs of drugs and related supplies.[19] In essence, these instructions allowed for payment of no more than the going rate for prescription drugs, and encouraged providers to minimize pharmacy costs "by obtaining discounts, either direct or indirect, from the supplier." These instructions also allowed for a separate pharmacist's fee for consultant and drug monitoring services.

The instructions further elaborate on the consultant fee:

"The charge for consultant services may be included in the provider's administrative costs, to the extent reasonable. The provider should document the extent of these services received so that any payment for them may be evaluated under the prudent buyer policy. It is recognized, however, that in many cases it would not be reasonable to charge the provider for the services, since the pharmacist already receives compensating value in the volume of prescription business done under the arrangement with the provider."

In June 1977, the federal Medicaid guidelines for reimbursement for pharmacy consultant services were released.[20] These guidelines advocate reimbursement for pharmacy consultant services: "This service is a cost of operation and is an allowable cost to the facility calculating the reimbursement rate from the State."

Some state Medicaid programs, even before release of the federal reimbursement guidelines, provided for reimbursement to the pharmacist for consultant and drug monitoring services. Effective October 1, 1974, Idaho's program began paying $10 per hour or $2 per patient per month, whichever is less. California, as of July 13, 1975 began paying 6.16 cents per patient per day. New Jersey, for a number of years, even prior to the new regulations, has paid 5 cents per patient per day.[21] Nevada pays 10 cents per patient per day up to a limit of the equivalent of $10 per hour.[22] In Massachusetts, 6 cents per patient day was added to nursing home rates effective January 1, 1977, for consultant and drug monitoring services, but only after a concerted effort by the state pharmaceutical association. The state association retained an attorney who reminded the State Rate Setting Commission that Section 1902(a)(13)(E) of the Social Security Act required payment to skilled nursing and intermediate care facilities on a reasonable cost "related" basis.[23]

Even though five states have formally recognized consultant and drug monitoring services in their reimbursement rates, pharmacists still protest that this compensation does not reach them. At one time, this complaint prompted the federal Medicaid program to issue the following draft reimbursement guidance: on premises observation of patients, nursing notes, laboratory reports, and drug administration records are necessary. Moreover, an on-premise individual medication record (drug profile) for all patients, not just 14 percent, is necessary to conduct such reviews.

Although insufficient time had elapsed for attaining full compliance with the drug regimen review requirement, these data were cause for concern that altruism and the opportunity to fulfill a clinical drug monitoring function alone would not be sufficient incentive to sustain this important patient care activity.

"Consulting pharmacists often complain that although the facility is reimbursed for the cost of pharmacy consultant services, the nursing home operator does not compensate the pharmacist for his consultant services. In such cases, the consultant pharmacist is also the prime vendor of prescribed drugs in the facility and the operator expects him to furnish consultant services free in exchange for getting the prescription business. This is illegal, and both the pharmacist and the facility operator are subject to Federal penalties up to $10,000 fine or a year in prison or both."[24]

## Monitoring to Reduce Prescriptions

One of the key objectives of monthly drug regimen reviews in skilled nursing facilities is the reduction, subject to the approval of attending physicians, in unwarranted or unnecessary drugs. Such reductions decrease patient exposure to unneeded drugs and, therefore, to unnecessary risks. One of the first investigations into the importance of this objective was conducted in 1972 by Cheung and Kayne[25] in southern California. Their study of 517 patients showed that a pharmacist could appropriately reduce the average number of prescriptions per patient per month from 6.8 to 5.6.

In another report by Rawlings and Frisk[26] on a four-year study of 260 patients, a prescription per patient per month average reduction of 7.7 to 6.1 was realized and the authors attribute this reduction to "effective automatic stop order policy, and careful review of patients' medication profiles by the pharmacists." Subsequently in 1974, Hood[27] and his coworkers conducted a study of 40 long-term care facility patients in Florida and showed that a reduction of 7.6 to 6.7 prescriptions could be appropriately realized. In an unpublished study by Marttila,[28] the drug regimens of 20 randomly selected patients were analyzed before and after drug monitoring was instituted in December 1976. The results of this Minnesota study showed an appropriate reduction of drug orders from 7.2 to 5.6.

An almost concurrent study was conducted in Northern California by Lofholm[29] in a 55-bed facility. This 13-month drug monitoring program resulted in an average monthly prescription reduction of 6.8 to 4.6 per patient. The most recent study was conducted by Cooper and Bagwell.[30] In this as yet unpublished one-year study, concluded in August 1977, changes in drug use of 142 patients resulted in an appropriate reduction of 7.22 to 4.78 prescriptions per patient.

These studies, in widely separated parts of the country, conducted by different pharmacists in different facilities, staffed by different nursing and medical personnel, demonstrate the wisdom of the skilled nursing facility regulation requiring drug monitoring by the pharmacist. Moreover, these studies provide considerable evidence that such monitoring can provide recommendations to physicians that appropriately reduce drug utilization in the range of 0.9 prescriptions per patient per month (Hood) to 2.44 prescriptions per patient per month (Cooper and Bagwell). The most frequent reduction would probably be about 1.5 prescriptions per patient per month (Cheung and Kayne: 1.2; Rawlings and Frisk: 1.6; Marttila: 1.6; and Lofholm: 2.2).

## Potential Cost Savings

Because these studies were conducted under widely differing geographic and other circumstances, one could infer that average reductions of the same magnitude can be realized for all skilled nursing facility patients. Moreover, it is reasonable to assume that the average quantity of a prescription drug order is equivalent to a month's drug supply. Thus, for each skilled nursing facility patient month, the price of one prescription can potentially be saved as a result of drug regimen reviews. Using the 0.9 prescriptions per patient per month reduction, the gross nationwide saving to the Medicare and Medicaid programs could amount to approximately $19.8 million per year.[c] Using the 2.44 prescription reduction figure, the gross nationwide saving could amount to approximately $53.8 million per year.

The cost of performing these reviews is reported to be 13 cents[31] and 14.37 cents[32] per patient per day. If one uses an upper limit of 15 cents per patient day, the monthly cost is approximately $4.50, and the annual nationwide cost of pharmacy consultant services, including the drug regimen reviews, amounts to approximately $16.6 million.[d]

Subtracting the cost of performance of these reviews from the gross savings, yields net savings to the Medicare and Medicaid programs of $3.2 million per year for the 0.9 prescription per month reduction, and $37.2 million per year for the 2.44 prescription reduction. It is reasonable to infer that savings of this magnitude could be realized if the drug regimen of every skilled nursing facility patient were adequately reviewed by pharmacists. If the same monitoring process were applied to intermediate care facility patients, an additional net savings ranging from $3.5 to $40.9 million could be realized.[e]

## Other Cost Considerations

This analysis describes only savings resulting from the reduction in *unwarranted* or *unnecessary drugs.* Cost savings that can result from a reduced rate of hospitalization caused by inappropriate drug therapy are not as easily documented. However, a recent study by Morse and LeRoy[33] provides good insight into the magnitude of these savings. In their 1977 study of nine hospitals equally distributed demographically within and between California, Arkansas and Minnesota, a total of 9,117 hospital admissions were examined.

Using conservative criteria for what constitutes "inappropriate drug therapy," these investigators documented 489 admissions that had a high probability of being drug induced. Of the 489 admissions, 113 or 23 percent were formerly skilled nursing facility patients. The authors conservatively estimate that the hospitalization of 45 of these patients could have been avoided with a minimal level of drug review, and that the "avoidable" hospitalizations resulted in expenditures of $53,000 for the Medicaid program alone.[34] (Medicare cross-over expenditures were undeterminable.)

Other evidence of reduced hospital cost comes from a 1972 study by Cheung and Kayne.[35] In their work with 517 patients, an estimated 68 hospitalizations were avoided when adverse drug reactions were detected through drug regimen reviews. The authors estimated that these hospitalizations could have

resulted in expenditures of $49,000.

While the results of these studies probably cannot reasonably be projected to all Medicare and Medicaid hospital admissions, they do provide good evidence that such savings can be realized, and that such savings are *in addition* to savings accomplished through the appropriate reduction in average monthly prescriptions per patient.

## Quality Considerations

Monetary improvements are only a part of the value that could be realized from the government's drug regimen review requirement. Quality considerations such as reduction in medication errors and reduction in inappropriate drug therapy have a profound but largely unquantifiable effect on patient well being and rehabilitation. Vlasses[36] has shown that 71 percent (10 out of 14) of his drug-related recommendations; 58 percent (37 out of 63) of his disease related recommendations; and 90 percent (10 out of 11) of his administrative recommendations, were approved by the attending physicians.

In the study by Cheung and Kayne,[37] 122 potential adverse drug reactions were detected and prevented. Sixty-eight of these reactions were considered clinically significant enough potentially to require hospitalization. In addition, this study showed that drug monitoring activities of a pharmacist reduced the medication administration error rate from 20 percent to 8 percent. The Hood[38] study also showed that 88 percent (15 out of 17) of the recommendations for improving drug therapy were accepted and acted on by attending physicians, and all 23 recommendations made to nursing personnel were accepted and implemented.

This information, plus the fact that all reductions in average monthly prescription utilization were accomplished with the approval of the attending physicians, attests to the fact that the quality of drug therapy and therefore patient care is enhanced through pharmacists' drug regimen reviews.

## Kickbacks: The Antithesis of Quality

An invidious kickback problem has seriously infected and retarded the advancement of quality pharmaceutical services in nursing homes. The kickback problem has been the subject of repeated congressional inquiries,[39 40 41] is rooted to a considerable extent in the practice of allowing volume discounts, and is causing serious adverse consequences for the patient.

Discounts from pharmacists to nursing homes probably began as legitimate arrangements in return for a larger volume of prescription business. However, over the years discounts have acted to increase program costs and reduce quality of care. Discounts have affected competition so as to drive many pharmacists away from nursing home service,[42] leaving the business to the "highest" discount bidder[43] who, through various means[44] [f] passes these additional costs on to the Medicare and Medicaid programs. It has been estimated that discounts given by pharmacists could amount to as much as $80 million.[45] If these discounts are not passed on to Medicare and Medicaid, as might be the case during difficult economic times, they become kickbacks.

The net effect of tolerating discounts in the

pharmacy-nursing home field is higher, not lower, public outlays, and because discounts are good precursors to kickbacks, an exacerbation of the kickback problem.

Discounts even when they do not become kickbacks are in and of themselves antithetical to quality drug therapy, given present requirements for drug regimen reviews. This is because the very basis of discounts is increased volume of prescription business. But the performance of drug regimen reviews has as a basic objective the reduction of unnecessary or unwarranted drugs, and therefore the reduction of prescription volume. Thus, if a discount is paid in order to gain prescription volume, one would want to maintain that volume—not reduce it—through the performance of in-depth drug regimen reviews.

Other evidence that the discount/kickback problem is harmful to quality of care comes from reports[46] that some nursing homes have guaranteed a specific volume of prescriptions per month for a return of 50 cents per prescription. This practice could expose the patient to unnecessary drug therapy, unnecessary risks and therefore poor quality. Most distressing is the reported practice of providing consultant and drug monitoring services free of charge.

A congressional report emphasizes the problems of this practice. In the words of the report: "Since these activities include reviewing a patient's drug regimen and reporting any medical irregularities, penetrating questions are raised as to whether illegal kickback arrangements are having an adverse effect on the health care of patients. This situation should be particularly questioned when a pharmacist is required to provide any nondispensing or quality review services 'free'."[47] This statement emphasizes that "free arrangements," whether termed discounts or kickbacks, for the most part can result only in cursory drug regimen reviews. Such reviews, as evidenced by drug reduction evidence brought together in this paper, can represent a significant detriment to the quality of care.

As HEW and states intensify their anti-fraud and abuse activities, the kickback situation will hopefully be minimized. The government's ability to cope with the kickback situation has, however, been compromised to a considerable extent by its past and present tolerance of discounts to nursing homes for pharmaceutical services. As these services have become less product-oriented and more patient-oriented, discounts/kickbacks have become a much greater detriment to the quality of drug therapy the patient receives.

## Conclusion

The information brought together in this paper provides strong evidence that drug regimen reviews performed by pharmacists for long-term care facility patients represent a significant opportunity to improve the quality of nursing home care, and do so at a net savings to the taxpayer. There is, however, some danger that this opportunity may be lost because of unenlightened reimbursement policies and "free-service arrangements." A pharmacist, or any other provider of a service, will not wholeheartedly engage in an activity for which there is no compensation—regardless of whether that lack of compensation is due to inadequate or nonexistent third party reimbursement, or to "free service arrangements" offered for, or solicited

in the name of, additional prescription volume. This is especially true if that activity is likely to reduce prescription volume and thus income.

Unless there is greater public recognition of the value of nursing home drug monitoring services in terms of reimbursement, in terms of regulation enforcement, and in terms of kickback deterrence, it is likely that the "paper consultant" will soon again prevail, and once again "over-drugging" and "medication errors" will be the subject of congressional reports. But worst of all, it is likely that the patient will not receive the quality of drug therapy that is attainable and very likely attainable at a net savings to the public.

*Samuel W. Kidder, PharmD, MPH, is a program analyst with the Division of Health Protection, Office of Health Policy, Research and Statistics, Office of the Assistant Secretary for Health, Department of Health, Education and Welfare. In this paper Dr. Kidder is writing in a private capacity, and no official support or endorsement by HEW or any of its agencies or offices is intended or should be inferred.*

a. The American Pharmaceutical Association, the American Society of Hospital Pharmacists and the American Nursing Home Association cooperated in the development of *Pharmaceutical Services in the Nursing Home*. The first edition of this document in 1963 could be viewed as the first pharmacy standards for this practice setting.

b. Even though these regulations changed the pharmacist's role by emphasizing a staff responsibility for drug monitoring services, the term "consultant pharmacist" remains in common usage. The term "non-dispensing services" is also used to describe these services, but less frequently. This author prefers the terminology "consultant and drug monitoring services" because it lends proper emphasis to the drug regimen review function.

c. This figure is based on the reduction in prescriptions per patient per month, times the number of reimbursed months of Medicare and Medicaid skilled nursing care, times the 1977 average prescription price of $5.98 as reported by International Medical Systems of America. The number of Medicare patient months was calculated from 1976 covered days of care available from the Office of Policy Planning and Research, Health Care Financing Administration, HEW. The number of Medicaid patient months was calculated from days of care obtained from *State Tables Fiscal Year 1975, Medicaid: Recipients, Payments and Services*; Health Care Financing Administration, Office of Policy, Planning and Research, Office of Research. Fiscal year 1975 data were used for all states except Connecticut and Arkansas (1974 data), Pennsylvania (1973 data) and Rhode Island, New York and Colorado (1972 data). Data for Maine, North Carolina and Arizona were not available in any recent year.

d. Calculated by multiplying $4.50 per month times the number of covered months of Medicare and Medicaid skilled nursing facility care using the same reporting years as was used for calculating potential savings.

e. Calculated from 1975 Medicaid data available from *Medicaid Recipient Characteristics and Units of Selected Medical Services, Fiscal Year 1975*. These data exclude information from Connecticut, Rhode Island, New York, Pennsylvania, Arkansas, Colorado, Maine, North Carolina, and Arizona.

f. For example: billing welfare departments for nonexistent prescriptions; supplying generic drugs and charging the state for brand name drugs; dispensing less than the prescribed amount and billing for the full amount; and billing for refills not dispensed.

# References

1. Griffenhagen, G. B., "Editorial—The Ever-Whirling Wheel of Change," *J. Am. Pharm. Assn., NS6*, 235(1966).

2. McLeod, D. C. and F. M. Eckel, "Reimbursement and Scope of Pharmacy Service in Nursing Homes, *J. Am. Pharm. Assn., NS9*, 62(1969).

3. Calculated from *Medicare: Use of Skilled Nursing Facility Services* 1969-73, H1-75 Feb. 2, 1977, Table 4, Page 8; Social Security Administration, Office of Program Policy and Planning, Office of Research and Statistics.

4. *Ibid.*, Table 4, p. 8.

5. *Trends in Long Term Care*, Hearings before the Subcommittee on Long Term Care of the Special Committee on Aging, United States Senate. Part 11—Washington, D.C., December 17, 1970, Statement by the National Council of Health Care Services, p. 971.

6. Congressional Record—Senate, *Tranquilizers—Largest Drug Category in Nursing Homes*, September 13, 1971, pp. 14170-14172.

7. Magnus, A. B., "Tranquilizers in Nursing Homes? A Question of Use, Abuse, or Misuse, *Nursing Homes*, July 1972, pp. 31-33.

8. Magnus, A. B., "Are Tranquilizers Used as "Chemical Straight Jackets"? Do Adequate Safeguards Exist?," *Nursing Homes*, March 1972, p. 24.

9. Congressional Record—Senate, *Medicaid Drugs in Nursing Homes*, April 27, 1972, pp. 6855-6860.

10. *Op. cit., Trends in Long Term Care* Part 11—Washington, D.C., December 17, 1970, p. 912.

11. General Accounting Office, *Continuing Problems in Providing Nursing Home Care and Prescribed Drugs Under the Medicaid Program in California*, 1970, p. 19.

12. *Drugs in Nursing Homes; Misuse, High Costs, and Kickbacks*; Subcommittee on Long Term Care of the Special Committee on Aging, United States Senate, January 1975.

13. "Report of Task Force on the Pharmacist's Clinical Role," *J. Am. Pharm. Assn., NS11*, September 1971.

14. Department of Health, Education, and Welfare, Health Resources Administration, Bureau of Health Manpower, Health Professions Schools, Selected BHM Support Data FY1965-76, December 1977 DHEW Publication No. (HRA) 78-37.

15. *Federal Register*, Vol. 39, No. 12, Thursday, January 17, 1975, pp. 2238-2257.

16. *Long-Term Care Facility Improvement Study, Introductory Report*, July 1975, Department of Health, Education, and Welfare, Public Health Service, Office of Nursing Home Affairs DHEW Publication No. (OS) 76-50021.

17. Contract No. HSM 110-73-421 "Pharmacy Training for Nursing Homes", American Pharmaceutical Association, Samuel H. Kalman, Project Director.

18. *Op. cit., Long-Term Care Facility Improvement Study, Introductory Report* July 1975, pp. 54, 56.

19. Department of Health, Education, and Welfare, Social Security Administration, *Medicare Provider Reimbursement Manual Revision*, Part I, HIM 15-1 October 1975, No. 134, Section 2103.1 Rev. 134.

20. Department of Health, Education, and Welfare, Health Care Financing Administration, *Medical Assistance Manual* Part 6 General Program Administration, 6-160-00, Reasonable Charges for Prescribed Drugs, p. 36.

21. Kidder, S. W., "Skilled Nursing Facilities—A Clinical Opportunity for Pharmacists, *Am. J. Hosp. Pharm., 34*, 751(1977).

22. ASCP UPDATE, American Society of Consultant Pharmacists, September 1977.

23. Simons, J. H., "Reimbursement of Pharmacy Consultant Services—A Case Study," *The Apothecary*, Sept/Oct 1977.

24. *Op. cit., Medical Assistance Manual*, p. 36.

25. Cheung, A. and R. Kayne, "An Application of Clinical Pharmacy Services for Extended Care Facilities," *Calif. Pharm.*, September 1975, p. 22.

26. Rawlings, J. L. and P. A. Frisk, "Pharmaceutical Services for Skilled Nursing Facilities in Compliance with Federal Regulations," *Am. J. Hosp. Pharm., 32*, 905(1975).

27. Hood, J. C. *et al.*, "Promoting Appropriate Therapy in a Long-Term Care Facility," *J. Am. Pharm. Assn., NS15*, January 1975.

28. Unpublished study by Dr. James K. Marttila, Pharmaceutical Consultant Services, Inc., 2675 University Ave., Hubbard Building #102, St. Paul, MN 55114, (612) 645-2139

29. Brodie, D. C. *et al.*, "A Model for Drug Use Review in a Skilled Nursing Facility," *J. Am. Pharm. Assn., NS17*, October 1977.

30. Cooper, J. W. and C. G. Bagwell. Presented to the Ninth Annual Regional Conference for Hospital Pharmacy Teachers, Residents and/or Graduate Students, University of Georgia, Athens, Georgia, Jan. 14, 1978. Submitted for publication to the *Journal of American Geriatrics Society*, and in review.

31. Vlasses, P. H. *et al.*, "Drug Therapy in a Skilled Nursing Facility: An Innovative Approach," *J. Am. Pharm. Assn., NS17*, February 1977.

32. Testimony presented at the California Department of Health Public Hearings, Sept. 23, 1976, by Dr. Ronald Kayne, Director of Education, California Pharmaceutical Association.

33. Leroy, A. A. and M. L. Morse, *A Study of the Impact of Inappropriate Ambulatory Drug Therapy on Hospitalization*; Contract No. NCFA-500-770011, Department of Health, Education, and Welfare, Health Care Financing Administration.

34. Personal Communication with M. Lee Morse, President, Health Information Designs Inc., 1629 K St., N.W., Suite 701, Washington, DC 20006, (202) 296-1934.

35. *Op. cit.*, Cheung, A. and R. Kayne, p. 28.

36. *Op. cit.*, Vlasses *et al.*, p. 93.

37. *Op. cit.*, Cheung, A. and R. Kayne, p. 24.

38. *Op. cit.*, Hood *et al.*, Calculated from Table II.

39. Hearings of the Subcommittee on Medicare and Medicaid of the Senate Finance Committee, June 16, 1970.

40. *Op. cit., Drugs in Nursing Homes: Misuse, High Costs, and Kickbacks*, January 1975.

41. *Fraud and Abuse in Nursing Homes: Pharmaceutical Kickback Arrangements* Subcommittee on Oversight and Investigations of the Committee on Interstate and Foreign Commerce, House of Representatives, March 1977.

42. *Ibid.*, p. 19.

43. *Ibid.*, p. 19.

44. *Op. cit., Drugs in Nursing Homes: Misuse, High Costs and Kickbacks*, January 1975, p. 290.

45. Hearings of the Subcommittee on Medicare and Medicaid of the Senate Finance Committee, June 16, 1970.

46. *Op. cit., Fraud and Abuse in Nursing Homes: Pharmaceutical Kickback Arrangements* March 1977, p. 20.

47. *Ibid.*, p. 27.

# VII.   Manufacturers and Suppliers of LTCF Materials

Abbott Laboratories
Pharmaceutical Products Division
14th and Sheridan Road, D-355
North Chicago, IL 60064
(312) 688-0322
- *Medications in unit dose packages*

Acme Visible Records, Inc.
Crozet, VA 22932
(804) 823-4351
- *Distribution and storage equipment*
- *Patient record systems*

Adhere Products
871 Redna Terrace
Cincinnati, OH 45215
(513) 771-8710
- *Patient record systems*
- *Printing and labeling equipment*
- *Health care identification systems*

Akro-Mils
1293 South Main Street
Akron, OH 44309
(216) 253-5592
- *Distribution and storage equipment*

Allergan Pharmaceuticals, Inc.
2525 Dupont Drive
Irvine, CA 92713
(714) 833-8880
- *Medications in unit dose packages*

American College of Apothecaries
874 Union Avenue, Room 9
Memphis, TN 38163
(901) 528-6037
- *Patient record systems*

Arenco Machine Company, Inc.
500 Hollister Road
Teterboro, NJ 07608
(201) 288-4444
- *Injectable filling equipment and supplies*
- *Filling, stoppering, and capping*
- *Tube filling*

Armour Pharmaceutical Company
Greyhound Tower
111 West Clarendon Avenue
Phoenix, AZ 85077
(602) 248-2820
- *Medications in unit dose packages*

Associated Bag Company
160 South Second Street
Milwaukee, WI 53204
(414) 272-2380
- *Unit dose*
- *Press on filing pockets, etc.*
- *Poly can liners, color-coded bags, plastic gloves, aprons*

Automated Packaging Systems, Inc.
8400 Darrow Road
Twinsburg, OH 44087
(216) 425-4242
- *Medications in unit dose packages*
- *Printing and labeling equipment*

Automated Prescription Systems, Inc.
P.O. Box 868
Pineville, LA 71360
(318) 445-7179
- *Outpatient or individual orders*

ASCO
Executive Offices, 2nd floor
8561 Fenton Street
Silver Spring, MD 20910
(301) 588-5800
- *Distribution and storage equipment*
- *Unit dose systems . . . complete*
- *Patient record systems*
- *Controlled substances counting, control system*

Avery Label
777 E. Foothill Blvd.
Azusa, CA 91702
(213) 969-3311
- *Printing and labeling equipment*

The Baker Company, Inc.
P.O. Drawer E—Sanford Airport
Sanford, ME 04073
(207) 324-8773
- *Laminar flow cabinets*

Briggs/Will Ross, Inc.
7887 University, P.O. Box 1698
Des Moines, IA 50306
(515) 274-9221
- *Distribution and storage equipment*
- *Patient record systems*
- *Pharmacy-related pressure sensitive tapes and labels*

ChaRx Prescription Profile Co.
1812 Monterey Avenue
Berkeley, CA 94707
(415) 687-0515 or (415) 526-3686
- *Distribution and storage equipment*
- *Patient record systems*

Cozzoli Machine Company
401 East Third Street
Plainfield, NJ 07060
(201) 757-2040
- *Injectable filling equipment and supplies*
- *Unit dose*

Dallas Label and Box Company
2655 Freewood
Dallas, TX 75220
(214) 357-9201
- *Unit dose*
- *Patient record systems*
- *Printing and labeling equipment*
- *All labels, vials, reclosable, poly bags*

Datapos Division of Retailer Services
The Henry B. Gilpin Co.
901 Southern Avenue
Washington, DC 20032
(301) 630-4500
- *Stand alone in store pharmacy computer systems*

Drug Package, Inc.
Medi-Aid Systems
O'Fallon, MO 63366
(314) 272-6261
- *Distribution and storage equipment*
- *Unit dose*
- *Patient record systems*
- *Labels*

Drustar Inc.
Brooknam Drive
Grovecity, OH 43123
(614) 875-1056 OH, (800) 848-0403 Toll Free
- *Distribution and storage equipment*
- *Unit dose*
- *Patient record systems*
- *Printing and labeling equipment*
- *U/D computer billing computerized patients charting records*

Dymo Visual Systems, Inc.
P.O. Box 1568
Augusta, GA 30903
(404) 733-1012
- *Printing and labeling equipment*

Dynalab Corporation
P.O. Box 112
Rochester, NY 14601
(716) 334-2060
- *Distribution and storage equipment*
- *Injectable filling equipment and supplies*
- *Packaging equipment and system*
- *Printing and labeling equipment*

Elkins-Sinn, Inc.
2 Esterbrook Lane, P. O. Box 5483
Cherry Hill, NJ 08034
(609) 424-3700
- *Injectable filling equipment and supplies*
- *Medications in unit dose packages*

Equipto
225 S. Highland
Aurora, IL 60507
(312) 859-1000
- *Distribution and storage equipment*

Errich International Corporation
721 Broadway
New York, NY 10003
(212) 674-5252
- *Packaging equipment and system*

Ferndale Laboratories Inc.
780 E. Eight Mile Road
Ferndale, MI 48220
(313) 548-0900
- *Medications in unit dose packages*
- *Unit dose liquid medications*

Fidelity Products Company
705 Pennsylvania Avenue South
Minneapolis, MN 55426
(612) 540-9700 or (800) 328-0624
- *Distribution and storage equipment*

E. Fougera & Co.
Division of Byk-Gulden, Inc.
Hicksville, NY 11802
- *Medications in unit dose packages*

Geigy Pharmaceuticals
556 Morris Avenue
Summit, NJ 07901
(201) 277-5390
- *Medications in unit dose packages*

General Equipment Manufacturers
P.O. Box 836
Crystal Springs, MS 39059
(601) 892-2731
- *Distribution and storage equipment*

L. C. Gess, Inc.
5235 Tractor Road
Toledo, OH 43612
(419) 476-9586
- *Injectable filling equipment and supplies*
- *Medications in unit dose packages*
- *Unit dose*
- *Printing and labeling equipment*

Grand Rapids Sectional Equipment Co.
P.O. Box 6306
Grand Rapids, MI 49506
(616) 243-4963
- *Distribution and storage equipment*

Healthmark Industries
17006 Mack
Grosse Pointe, MI 48224
(313) 886-1753
- *Distribution and storage equipment*

Hodge Mfg. Co., Inc.
55 Fisk Ave.
Springfield, MA 01101
(413) 781-6800
- *Distribution and storage equipment*

Hoechst-Roussel Pharmaceuticals Inc.
RTS 202-206N
Somerville, NJ 08876
(201) 685-2858
- *Medications in unit dose packages*
- *Educational material*

Howard Sales, Inc.
2225 Belt Line Road, #106
P.O. Box 935
Carrollton, TX 75006
(214) 242-2138
- *Printing and labeling equipment*

Hynson, Westcott & Dunning, Inc.
Charles & Chase Streets
Baltimore, MD 21201
(301) 837-0890
- *Medications in unit dose packages*
- *Diagnostic health care products*

Inolex Medical Products Division of
Inolex Corporation Subsidiary of
American Can Company
3 Science Road
Glenwood, IL 60425
(312) 755-2933
- *Medications in unit dose packages*

Insta-Systems Co. Inc.
9911 Indian Queen Point Road
Oxon Hill, MD 20022
  • *Stand-alone in store pharmacy system*

Invenex Pharmaceuticals
5885 Lakehurst Drive
Orlando, FL 32805
(305) 351-1400
  • *Injectable medications in unit dose packages*

Ivers-Lee, Div. of Becton, Dickinson & Company
147 Clinton Road
West Caldwell, NJ 07006
(201) 575-9000
  • *Unit dose*

KCL Corporation
P.O. Box 629
Shelbyville, IN 46176
(317) 392-2521 & (800) 428-5431
  • *Unit dose*

Kewaunee Scientific Equipment Corp.
P.O. Drawer 5400
Statesville, NC 28677
(704) 873-7202
  • *Distribution and storage equipment*

Kole Enterprises, Inc.
3553 N.W. 50 St., (P.O. Box 520152)
Miami, FL 33152
(800) 327-6085, Fla. Residents call collect
(305) 633-2556
  • *Distribution and storage equipment*

Labelon Corporation
10 Chapin Street
Canandiaqua, NY 14424
(716) 394-6220
  • *Patient record systems*
  • *Labels*

Lederle Labs.
N. Middletown Road
Pearl River, NY 10965
(914) 735-5000
  • *Medications in unit dose packages*

LEWISystems/Menasha Corp.
426 Montgomery Street
Watertown, WI 53094
(414) 261-3162
  • *Distribution and storage equipment*

Eli Lilly and Company
307 E. McCarty Street
Indianapolis, IN 46206
(317) 636-2211
  • *Medications in unit dose packages*

Lynn Peavey Company
15551 W. 109th St.—P.O. Box 5555
Lenexa, KS 66215
(913) 888-0600
  • *Reclosable poly bags for pharmacy use*

Macbick Div. D. R. Bard Inc.
111 Spring Street
Murray Hill, NJ 07974
(201) 277-8000
  • *Distribution and storage equipment*
  • *Carts*

Mallinckrodt, Inc.
Pharmaceutical Products Division
675 Brown Road, P.O. Box 5840
St. Louis, MO 63134
(314) 895-0317
  • *Medications in unit dose packages*

Markem Corporation
150 Congress Street
Keene, NH 03431
(603) 352-1130
  • *Printing and labeling equipment*

Market Forge
35 Garvey Street
Everett, MA 02149
(617) 387-4100
  • *Distribution and storage equipment*

Material Handling Division
Midland Ross Corp.
10605 Chester Road
Cincinnati, OH 45215
(513) 772-1313/(800) 543-4454
  • *Distribution and storage equipment*

McNeil Laboratories
500 Office Center Drive
Fort Washington, PA 19034
(215) 628-5000
  • *Medications in unit dose packages*

Mead Johnson Pharmaceutical Division
2404 Pennsylvania Street
Evansville, IN 47721
(812) 426-7069
  • *Medications in unit dose packages*

Medical Packaging Inc.
525 Whitehorse Pike
Atco, NJ 08004
(609) 767-3604
  • *Distribution and storage equipment*
  • *Injectable filling equipment and supplies*
  • *Unit dose solid and liquid*

Medi-Dose, Inc.
1671 Loretta Avenue
Feasterville, PA 19047
(215) 322-7555
  • *Medications in unit dose packages*
  • *Medi-Dose/Medi-Cup system in house manual, extemporaneous unit-dose packaging*
  • *Printing and labeling equipment*
  • *Wheaton medi-systems prescription vials*

Medipak, Inc.
P.O. Box 201
409 S. Illinois Street
Springfield, IL 62705
(217) 546-5131
  • *Distribution and storage equipment*
  • *Unit dose*
  • *Printing and labeling equipment*
  • *Out of pharmacy drug control system*

Merck Sharp & Dohme
West Point, PA 19486
(215) 699-5311
  • *Medications in unit dose packages*

Metropolitan Wire Corp.
N. Washington & George Aves.
Wilkes-Barre, PA 18705
(717) 825-2741
  • *Distribution and storage equipment*
  • *Unit dose*

Herman Miller, Inc.
Health/Science Division
8500 Byron Road
Zeeland, MI 49464
(616) 772-3322
  • *Distribution and storage equipment*

Modern Metals Industries, Inc.
128 Sierra Street, P.O. Box 888
El Segundo, CA 90245
(213) 322-6272/722-2881
  • *Medicine cart cassette cabinets, etc.*

Modern Office Devices, Inc.
731 Hempstead Turnpike
Franklin Square, NY 11010
(516) 483-9410
  • *Rx cabinets*
  • *Patient record systems*
  • *Labels*
  • *Rx balance, Rx glassware, data collection systems*

Monarch Marking Systems, Inc.
P.O. Box 608
Dayton, OH 45401
(513) 865-2123
  • *Printing and labeling equipment*
  • *Data collection systems*

Monarch Metal Products, Inc.
P.O. Box 4081
New Windsor, NY 12550
(914) 562-3100
  • *Carts for distribution of unit dose medications*

MPL, Inc.
SoloPak Division
1820 W. Roscoe
Chicago, IL 60657
(800) 621-6421/IL Call Collect (312) 248-3810
  • *Injectable filling equipment and supplies*
  • *Unit dose liquid*

National Instrument Company, Inc.
4119 Fordleigh Road
Baltimore, MD 21215
(301) 764-0900
  • *Injectable filling equipment and supplies*
  • *Liquid fillers, aluminum cap closers, screw cap tighteners, capsule fillers*

Norwich Eaton Pharmaceuticals
17 Eaton Avenue
Norwich, NY 13815
(607) 335-2111
  • *Medications in unit dose packages*

Organon Pharmaceuticals
375 Mt. Pleasant Avenue
West Orange, NJ 07052
(201) 325-4600
  • *Medications in unit dose packages*

Owens-Illinois
Prescription Products Div.
Post Office Box 1035
Toledo, OH 43666
(419) 247-0313
  • *Unit dose packaging and equipment*
  • *Prescription containers and closures*

Paco Packaging, Inc.
7401 Central Highway
Pennsauken, NJ 08109
(609) 662-0996 or (215) 922-2210
  • *Medications in unit dose packages*

Parke-Davis & Co.
UNI/USE Systems Division
208 Welsh Pool Road
Lionville, PA 19353
(215) 363-9100
  • *Distribution and storage equipment*
  • *Medications in unit dose packages*
  • *Unit dose*
  • *Patient record systems, nursing and pharmacy*
  • *Printing and labeling equipment*
  • *Distribution systems*

Perry Industries, Inc.
121 New South Road
Hicksville, NY 11802
(516) 433-2230
  • *Injectable filling equipment and supplies*
  • *Packaging equipment and system*

Pfipharmecs Division of Pfizer Pharmaceuticals
235 East 42nd Street
New York, NY 10017
(212) 573-2323
  • *Medications in unit dose packages*

Pharmacia Laboratories
800 Centennial Avenue
Piscataway, NJ 08854
(201) 469-1222 X209
  • *Medications in unit dose packages*

PharmAssist
1801 West Euless Blvd.
Euless, TX 76039
(817) 469-2428
- *Patient record systems*

Phenix Rx Supplies
4120 Pennsylvania
Kansas City, MO 64111
(816) 931-1766
- *Distribution and storage equipment*
- *Patient record systems*
- *Printing and labeling equipment*
- *Plastic containers, prescription boxes, pharmacy equipment*

Philips Roxane Laboratories, Inc.
330 Oak Street
Columbus, OH 43216
(614) 228-5403
- *Distribution and storage equipment*
- *Medications in unit dose packages*
- *Packaging equipment and system*
- *Printing and labeling equipment*

Physicians' Record Co.
3000 S. Ridgeland Ave.
Berwyn, IL 60402
(312) 749-3111
- *Distribution and storage equipment, boxes*
- *Patient record systems*
- *Printing and labeling equipment*
- *Lab requisitions and charge slips*

Presto-TEK Corporation
7321 N. Figueroa St.
Los Angeles, CA 90041
(213) 257-7585
- *Container and drum pumps, trigger sprayers, pH meters, colorimeters, dialysate test meters*

Production Equipment Inc.
17 Legion Place
Rochelle Park, NJ 07662
(201) 845-4475
- *Injectable filling equipment*
- *Tablet, capsule, liquid-bulk and unit dose*

Professional Tape Co., Inc.
144 Tower Dr.
Burr Ridge, IL 60521
(312) 986-1800
- *Printing and labeling equipment*

Prospect Park Press
P.O. Box 33—Farr Road
West Chesterfield, NH 03466
(603) 256-6372
- *Patient record systems*
- *General printing custom forms for medical field*

Pure-Aire Corporation
15544 Cabrito Road
Van Nuys, CA 91406
(213) 781-2201
- *Packaging equipment and system*
- *Laminar flow hoods*

Pyramid Products Corp.
31 B. Columbia Ave.
Philadelphia, PA 19125
(215) 426-0588
- *Folding boxes*

Quik Chek Systems Inc.
19189 W. Ten Mile Road
Southfield, MI 48075
(313) 358-4020
- *Patient record systems*

Reed & Carnrick
30 Boright Avenue
Kenilworth, NJ 07033
(201) 272-6600
- *Pharmaceuticals*

Respiratory Care Inc.
900 W. University Drive
Arlington Heights, IL 60004
(312) 259-7400
- *Unit dose*

A. H. Robins Company, Inc.
1407 Cummings Drive
Richmond, VA 23220
(804) 257-2215
- *Medications in unit dose packages*

Roche Laboratories
340 Kingsland Road
Nutley, NJ 07110
(201) 235-2304
- *Booklets and audio visual*

Roerig Division of Pfizer Pharmaceuticals
235 E. 42nd Street
New York, NY 10017
(212) 573-2323
- *Medications in unit dose packages*

RxCount Corporation
14129 Chadron Ave.
Hawthorne, CA 90250
(213) 676-7854
- *Prescription counters*

Safeguard Business Systems, Inc.
470 Maryland Drive
Fort Washington, PA 19034
(215) 643-4811
- *Patient record systems*

Samuels Products Inc.
3929 Virginia Ave.
Cincinnati, OH 45227
(513) 271-4545
- *Piggyback or computer labels*
- *Printing and labeling equipment*

Sandoz Pharmaceuticals
59 Route 10
East Hanover, NJ 07936
(201) 386-7914
- *Medications in unit dose packages*
- *Medicines in shelf packages and in ampuls*

# Appendix

The Sargent Co.
1730 I Avenue NE
Cedar Rapids, IA 52402
(319) 363-1302
• *Distribution and storage equipment*

Savage Laboratories
1000 Main Street
Missouri City, TX 77459
(713) 499-4547
• *Medications in unit dosage packages*

Scheck-Builders Products, Inc.
108 Wooster St.—3rd Floor
New York, NY 10012
(212) 226-5433
• *Distribution and storage equipment*
• *Injectable filling equipment and supplies*
• *Packaging equipment and system*

Schering Corporation
Galloping Hill Road
Kenilworth, NJ 07033
(201) 931-2900
• *Medications in unit dose packages*

Scrip Stat Division of Retailer Services
The Henry B. Gilpin Co.
901 Southern Ave.
Washington, DC 20032
(301) 630-4500
• *Patient record systems*

Searle Laboratories
Box 5110
Chicago, IL 60680
(312) 679-7700
• *Medications in unit dose packages*

Shaw-Clayton Plastics, Inc.
123 Carlos Drive
San Rafael, CA 94903
(415) 472-1522
• *Distribution and storage equipment*

Shell Container Inc.
342 Great Neck Road
Great Neck, NY 11021
(516) 466-4505
• *Distribution and storage equipment*
• *Medications in unit dose packages*

Simplex Filler Company
3490 Investment Blvd.
Hayward, CA 94545
(415) 785-8010
• *Injectable filling equipment and supplies*

Smith Kline and French Laboratories
1500 Spring Garden St.
Philadelphia, PA 19101
(215) 854-4000
• *Medications in unit dose packages*

Stat Systems
P.O. Box 15691
Charlotte, NC 28210
(704) 525-4196
• *Patient record systems*

Soabar Division, Avery International
7722 Dungan Road
Philadelphia, PA 19111
(215) 725-4700
• *Unit dose packaging and labeling*
• *Patient record systems*
• *Printing and labeling equipment*

Stuart Pharmaceuticals
411 Silverside Road
P.O. Box 751
Wilmington, DE 19897
(800) 441-7758 or 59
• *Medications in unit dose packages*

Tenney Engineering Co.
1090 Springfield Rd.
Union, NJ 07083
(201) 686-7870
• *Mfg. environmental, bio-medical electronic equipment*

Thatcher Plastic Packaging
E-210 Route 4
Paramus, NJ 07652
(201) 845-0190/(212) 935-1720
• *Plastic squeeze tubes, celo bands, plastic closures, PVC shrinkage tubing*

Trans-Aid Corporation
1609 E. Del Amo
Carson, CA 90746
(213) 774-7023
• *Distribution and storage equipment*
• *Patient record systems*
• *Carts*

Unit Dose Packaging
2005 Mt. Vernon Ave.
Pomona, CA 91768
(714) 623-0775
• *Medications in unit dose packages*
• *Contract unit dose packaging*

Uni-Script, Inc.
1601 S. Calhoun St.
Ft. Wayne, IN 46804
(219) 744-3168
• *Distribution and storage equipment*
• *Unit dose*
• *Patient record systems*
• *Printing and labeling equipment*

United Hospital Supply Corp.
1900 Bannard St.
Cinnaminson, NJ 08077
• *Distribution and storage equipment*
• *Patient record systems*
• *Printing and labeling equipment*
• *Dispensing medication carts*

USV Laboratories
One Scarsdale Road
Tuckahoe, NY 10707
(914) 779-6300
- *Medications in unit dose packages*

Vernitron Medical Products
5 Empire Blvd.
Carlstadt, NJ 07072
(201) 641-5500
- *Distribution and storage equipment,
  narcotic cabinets*
- *Patient record systems*
- *Vials, sterilizers*

Vertrod Corporation
2037 Utica Avenue
Brooklyn, NY 11234
(212) 241-8080
- *Heat sealers, impulse type*

Wallace Laboratories
Div. of Carter-Wallace Inc.
Half Acre Road
Cranbury, NJ 08512
(609) 655-1100
- *Medications in unit dose packages*

Waterloo Industries Inc.
300 Ansbrough Ave, P.O. Box 209
Waterloo, IA 50704
(319) 235-7131
- *Distribution and storage equipment*

Weber Marketing Systems
711 W. Algonquin Rd.
Arlington Heights, IL 60005
(312) 439-8500
- *Unit dose*
- *Printing and labeling equipment*

Wheaton Industries
Wheaton Ave.
Millville, NJ 08332
(609) 825-1400
- *Distribution and storage equipment*
- *Liquid dispensing systems, aluminum seal and
  unit-dose hand crimping equipment, automatic
  crimpers*
- *Laboratory glassware, apparatus and equipment*

Wrapade Machine Co. Inc.
189 Sargeant Ave.
Clifton, NJ 07013
(201) 773-6150
- *Form, fill, and seal, peal seal chevron catch
  cover packaging equipment*